Fariza Halimova

ADAPTATION OF NEW POPULATION

Fariza Halimova

ADAPTATION OF NEW POPULATION

Features of adaptive reactions of the body of the newcomer
population of the agro-industrial region

Imprint

Any brand names and product names mentioned in this book are subject to trademark, brand or patent protection and are trademarks or registered trademarks of their respective holders. The use of brand names, product names, common names, trade names, product descriptions etc. even without a particular marking in this work is in no way to be construed to mean that such names may be regarded as unrestricted in respect of trademark and brand protection legislation and could thus be used by anyone.

Cover image: www.ingimage.com

This book is a translation from the original published under ISBN 978-620-4-97889-5.

Publisher:
Sciencia Scripts
is a trademark of
Dodo Books Indian Ocean Ltd. and OmniScriptum S.R.L publishing group

120 High Road, East Finchley, London, N2 9ED, United Kingdom
Str. Armeneasca 28/1, office 1, Chisinau MD-2012, Republic of Moldova, Europe
Printed at: see last page
ISBN: 978-620-7-62307-5

Fariza Tursunbaevna Khalimova

ADAPTATION OF THE IMMIGRANT POPULATION

PECULIARITIES OF ADAPTIVE REACTIONS OF THE ORGANISM OF THE IMMIGRANT POPULATION OF THE AGRO-INDUSTRIAL REGION

CONTENTS.

INTRODUCTION

Relevance of the topic. The study of human adaptation to changed environmental conditions remains one of the most important directions of modern ecological physiology. It is known that the objective study of individual features of human adaptation capabilities, their classification and typification are important in theoretical and applied aspects - [68, 114, 2, 95, 35, 9, 124, 135, 136, 137, 138, 5, 6, 7, 3, 36, 80, 177, 189].

To date, the criteria for assessing and predicting the effectiveness of human adaptation to changed conditions with the specification of the optimal period of living in these conditions without damage to the state of the organism in accordance with individual characteristics have not been sufficiently developed. The identification of such criteria will undoubtedly make it possible to carry out a targeted selection of persons for various works in areas with high anthropotechnogenic load without damage to the state of health.

Increased rhythm of life, urbanization with its negative environmental consequences, radical socio-economic and political transformations have increased the load on life-supporting systems of the body - [4, 8, 140, 36, 80].

Human professional activity is largely associated not only with the impact on the body of physical stress and nervous-emotional tension, but also with unusual environmental factors affecting its general condition, well-being and performance. Such environmental factors are referred to extreme factors - extreme and harsh environmental conditions, inadequate to the innate and acquired properties of the body - [17, 2, 9, 85, 91, 137, 6, 61, 80, 145]. The action of unfavorable environmental factors make increased demands on the adaptive capabilities of a person and cause a significant restructuring of the vital activity of all systems of the organism, and under unfavorable conditions create preconditions for the development of pathology - [33, 67, 94, 14, 125, 127, 60, 5, 3, 154, 152]. Analysis of the identification of environmental factors on various functional indicators of body systems seems to be extremely important in connection with the significant growth of industrial production and intensive environmental pollution - [29, 8, 146, 147]. At present, it is generally recognized that there is a direct relationship between environmental indicators and human health - [30, 149, 164, 160].

In order to obtain comprehensive information about the state of the human body living in conditions with a high rank of anthropotechnogenic load, a comprehensive approach based on modern diagnostic methods is necessary, a special place in which is given to the biochemical method of research [83, 39, 103, 28, 31, 54, 54, 49, 41, 174, 175, 180, 187]. However, the use of biochemical methods of research in assessing the functional state of migrants living in conditions with different ranks of anthropotechnogenic load is significantly complicated due to the impossibility of blood collection from a vein and finger. This necessitates the study of other human biological fluids and the development of bloodless methods that are more suitable in real-life conditions. One of the most accessible for study is saliva, the quantitative and qualitative composition of which depends on the influence of various endogenous and exogenous influences on the organism - [44, 90, 57, 88, 41, 47, 1, 158, 177, 157, 157, 151, 167, 178, 173, 165, 182, 161].

In connection with the above-mentioned, it seems relevant to study the state of functional indicators and adaptation capabilities of the human organism in conditions with low and high rank of anthropotechnogenic load.

Chapter 1: LITERATURE REVIEW

1.1 Modern concepts of health, adaptation process and functional reserves of the organism

The change of ecologically habitual habitats places increased demands on human adaptive capabilities and causes a significant restructuring of the vital activity of all body systems, and under unfavorable conditions create preconditions for the development of pathology - [133, 33, 94, 17, 2, 108, 70, 61, 7, 135, 137, 139, 140, 138, 129, 11, 145, 189, 171]. Extreme exposures to the body affect adaptive mechanisms, resulting in adaptation. Stress - syndrome is an integral component of adaptation to all factors without exception. Its main content is excitation of higher vegetative centers and, as a consequence, activation of stress-realizing systems, the main component of which is sympathoadrenal. As a result, the effect of high concentrations of catecholamines and glucocorticoids is realized. Both of these factors have a wide range of action in the organism, the main feature of which is the mobilization of energy and structural resources of the organism - [106, 102, 96, 5, 6, 122, 19, 140, 138].

When a person moves from other climatogeographic zones of habitat, in particular from the countries of the near abroad to the regions of the Russian Federation, depending on the severity of anthropotechnogenic load, contributes to a sharp change in the level of regulation of a single homeostatic mechanism and eventually failure of adaptation.

Migrant persons living in the conditions of agro-industrial region with different ranks of anthropotechnogenic load, experience the impact of unusual environmental factors that have an unfavorable impact on his general condition, well-being and performance. Such environmental factors belong to extreme factors, i.e. extreme, harsh environmental conditions, inadequate to the innate and acquired properties of the organism - [69, 91, 36, 146, 147, 160]. Under such conditions, the equilibration of an integral organism with the external environment is achieved only with the economical functioning of neuroendocrine regulation of the systems responsible for adaptation.

Numerous studies have been conducted by various authors to identify the effect of certain environmentally unfavorable factors on the human body - [92, 87, 134, 23, 24, 70, 149, 164, 155].

However, not always the human organism exposed to ecopathogenic factors can fully realize adaptation, which is associated with the depletion of energy and structural resources of the organism.

In a situation where there is no possibility of realizing adaptation, there will be a disturbance of homeostasis, which constitutes the stimulus of stress. Under the action of any stress, including ecopathogenic factors, first of all there is an activation of the sympathoadrenal system - [98, 104, 118, 96, 116, 125, 40, 53, 80, 190, 172]. As a result of prolonged and intensive action of concentrations of catecholamines and glucocorticoids, a wide variety of injuries can occur, constituting the field of so-called stressor diseases, which occupy one of the main places in modern medicine - [94, 105, 141, 115, 124, 2, 14, 37, 70, 89, 16, 19, 158].

The totality of eco-pathogenic factors that act on a person living in a region with a high rank of anthropotechnogenic load, cause stress on the adaptation reserves of the organism, can lead to their depletion and, therefore, require careful study.

Thus, it is necessary to assess the level of health and reserve capabilities of persons living in the agro-industrial region with different ranks of anthropotechnogenic load in order to prevent the depletion of adaptive resources of the organism and the prevention of stress-related diseases. This indicates the importance of developing new, adequate methods of studying the human organism.

The Thirtieth World Health Assembly laid the foundation for achieving health for all and resolved that the primary objective of Governments and WHO is for all the world's inhabitants to attain a level of health that will enable them to live productive social and economic lives. In the light of this resolution, the study of health status and the quantification of health levels assume great importance as a prerequisite for the subsequent progress of society - [13, 67, 18, 26, 107, 139, 139, 140, 138, 138, 93, 7, 127, 175, 189].

The earlier we can diagnose conditions in the intermediate region between health and disease, the better the chances of maintaining full health and active human activity.

To take healthy people in his hands, to protect them from hereditary or threatening diseases, to prescribe them a proper way of life is honest and for the doctor is peaceful, because it is easier to prevent diseases than to cure them. And this is his first duty (M.Y. Mudrov)

It is known that the state of human health is largely determined by the ecological and physiological features of human adaptation to the sharply changing conditions of modern life. Taking care of people's health and well-being requires theoretical developments and deep scientific substantiation. Health improvement of the population is closely connected with the realization of health-improving and preventive measures, not only with the activity of medical institutions. Some aspects of these topical problems were the subject of this study.

The study of stress mechanism shows that stress, adaptation and health are dependent processes - [111, 32, 117, 38, 10, 6, 19, 138, 70, 175, 189, 171]. Exposure to stress can lead to an increase in the functional reserve of the organism, thereby increasing its health status. On the other hand, stress can lead to exhaustion of the body's systems and the emergence of prenosological states that progress to disease. The two outcomes when exposed to stress depend on the adaptive capacity of the organism, which is determined by its level of health. The task of researchers is to identify quantitative and qualitative criteria for assessing and predicting the phase of adaptation, the degree of resistance of the organism to stress with the subsequent determination of health levels.

From the many definitions of health given by Bykov A.T. et al. (2004), the following points emerge:

1. The end result of health is physical, mental and social well-being

2. Most definitions note that health is the state of being human

3. There is a direct correlation between the functional reserve of the organism, the expression of regulatory mechanisms and human health

4. Health is closely related to the adaptive capacity of the organism to changing environmental conditions

It follows from the above that the transition from health to disease occurs through a gradual decline in the human ability to adapt to changing environmental conditions with overstrain and disruption of regulatory mechanisms, which leads to changes in homeostasis and a decrease in the level of health. It should be noted that to date there is no universally accepted classification of health levels. The most all-encompassing classification is health levels by the degree of tension of regulatory mechanisms and functional reserve:

I. Individuals with satisfactory adaptation: a) optimal level of regulatory mechanisms; b) normal level of regulatory mechanisms.

II. Persons with insufficient or unsatisfactory adaptation (prenosological conditions): a) moderate tension of regulatory mechanisms; b) pronounced tension of regulatory mechanisms; c) overstrain of regulatory mechanisms.

III. Persons with disruption of adaptation, with premorbid conditions, acute and chronic diseases: a) with predominance of nonspecific changes; b) with predominance of specific changes.

The first group is characterized by the state of the organism with a sufficiently high functional reserve, in which the average fluctuation of psychophysiological, biochemical, genetic and other parameters of the organism are able to keep the living system within its morphofunctional optimum with the absence or minimally expressed tension of regulatory mechanisms. The second group is characterized by a state in which homeostasis maintenance occurs due to various degrees of expression of tension of regulatory mechanisms with increased activity of sympathoadrenal and other systems of the organism. The third group is characterized by a decrease in the functional capabilities of the organism with the manifestation of insufficiency of protective and adaptive mechanisms and the inability of the organism to provide optimal adequate to the changed environmental conditions regulation of functional systems.

Thus, the problem of preserving and restoring human health requires the development of a system for diagnosing the state of individual reserves of the organism and the search for means that contribute to their optimal correction.

Continuous growth of scientific and socio-political information, limited time for its processing, imperfect mode of labor and rest generate disharmony in the development of personality - [126, 123, 42, 120]. In conditions of disharmony of the ratio of parameters of physiological indicators under the action of excessive stress there are tension, overstrain and failure of adaptation processes depending on the degree of such disharmony - [75, 92, 121, 142, 135, 140]. In this regard, there is a need to develop criteria for assessing the level of psychoemotional stress under stress and timely diagnosis of its inadequate impact on the body.

It is known that stress-response is a necessary link in the formation of adaptation of the organism to environmental factors. However, in case of excessively intensive or prolonged stress-response adaptation is not formed, and stress-response leads to damage and disorders of the organism's function up to the development of a number of psychosomatic diseases. At the same time, persistent adequate adaptation to the action of any stress prevents damage and increases the body's resistance to stress - [137, 4, 6, 48, 127, 171, 189].

One of the key tasks of diagnostics of prenosological state and prognosis of health state, both individual and group, is to identify risk factors, which can be determined with the help of various tests of assessment of the functional state of the organism.

Any activity activates the mechanism of stress, which has the function of adaptation to the arising difficult situation. The action of stress can increase the functional reserve of the organism and the level of its health - in the expression of Sellier - this is eustress. In this case, the reaction of the organism proceeds without losses of the organism. On the other hand, stress can lead to exhaustion of the body systems, to the emergence of prenosological state, which can go into disease - this is dysstress. Two outcomes of stress action depend on the functional reserve of the organism, its level of health and adaptive capabilities - [111, 112, 189, 176].

Currently, three degrees of functional reserve can be distinguished. Adaptation occurs due to the mobilization of functional reserves of the organism and requires a certain tension of regulatory systems. The problem of adaptation is that the "price of adaptation" did not go beyond the individual "limit", that is, did not lead to overstrain and exhaustion of regulatory mechanisms, which ultimately contributes to a decrease in the level of health. It is known that adaptation changes under the action of any stress begin with a nonspecific reaction of mobilization of functional reserves due to activation of the stress-realizing system, the main link of which is the sympathoadrenal system. The state in which the nonspecific component of the general adaptation syndrome manifests itself in the form of varying degrees of stress of regulatory systems is called prenosological - [19, 25, 27], in which there is a decrease in the level of health and the organism is between norm and disease. Further action of stress in this situation leads to overstrain of regulatory mechanisms, a sharp decrease in functional reserve, unsatisfactory adaptation is noted. In this state, along with nonspecific changes are more significant specific changes on the part of individual organs and systems, that is, the initial phenomena of premorbid state are noted, when changes already indicate the type of probable pathology. Thus, the manifestations of disease, which is the result of adaptation failure, are preceded by prenosological and premorbid states - [16, 19], which are accompanied by a decrease in functional reserve and health level. At the first stages, this mechanism ensures the existence of the organism in new conditions, but it is energetically uneconomical and depends entirely on the functional reserve of the organism and its level of health. The greater the functional reserve of the organism and the higher the level of health, the greater the chances of the organism's transition to a more stable and reliable mechanism of long-term adaptation. That is, determining the adaptive capabilities of the organism, we give an assessment of health levels, which depends entirely on the functional reserve of the organism and determine its functional state.

The above shows that stress, adaptation and health are interdependent processes. Thus, the final result of stress and adaptive capabilities of a person is the level of his/her health.

One of the tasks of modern physiology of adaptation is the timely detection of pre- and premorbid state of the organism, accompanied by a sharp decrease in functional reserve and health level. At present, there is no generally accepted methodology for diagnostics of functional reserve, health level and adaptive capabilities to stress. One of the ways to solve this problem is to assess the violation or degree of stress of regulatory systems of the integral organism. In this regard, the results of integral assessment of regulatory mechanisms of blood pressure, which characterizes the state of the cardiovascular system, can be considered reliable objective criteria. The solution of the gap in this area is possible due to the study of beta-adrenergic reactivity of erythrocyte membrane, reflecting the degree of activity of the sympathoadrenal system. An objective assessment of the state of the holistic organism can be given by changing the concentration of electrolytes, glucose and cortisol in human saliva and the types of their dynamics.

1.2 Physiological methods of functional state assessment human organism in conditions with different ranks of anthropotechnogenic load

To assess the functional state of the human body under various stresses, biochemical methods of research are one of the objective methods. However, there are a number of difficulties associated with blood collection from the vein and finger. On the other hand, the increasing incidence of AIDS, hepatitis and other infectious diseases has made an attempt to study other human biological fluids and to develop bloodless methods that are more suitable in real-life conditions - [59, 41, 45, 57, 62, 152, 153].

Noskov V.B. et al. (1991) emphasize the priority in this direction biochemical study of saliva as a non-invasive, informative and non-labor-intensive method of early diagnosis of human health disorders. The use of such methods seems to be especially valuable in some specific types of activity: in mass preventive examinations, in the selection of healthy persons for work of specialized purpose, in the experimental study of adaptive reactions of the organism to extreme influences. In recent years, biochemical studies of saliva have been practiced quite widely in extreme physiology [56, 47, 42, 55, 191, 174, 151, 161, 173, 167].

McLean C. et al. in 1989 studied adrenocorticosteroids in mountaineers at an altitude of 4500 m. Based on the data obtained, the authors concluded that saliva studies are useful for non-invasive health monitoring during an expedition.

Saliva is one of the most accessible biological fluids for research. Its quantitative and qualitative composition depends on the influence of various endogenous and exogenous influences on the organism - [39, 174, 152]. There are many works by various authors in which saliva is subjected to a comprehensive study - [131, 15, 155, 154]. It should be noted that the composition of saliva depends on the methodological features of saliva collection (time of day, environmental conditions), on the functional state of the nervous system, hormonal activity of the pituitary and adrenal glands - [100]. Mixed saliva of parotid, submandibular and hyoid glands consists of 99.5% water and 0.5% dry residue. Inorganic components of saliva are phosphorus, calcium, potassium, sodium, magnesium, fluorine, iodine, nickel and other elements - [84].

Of organic substances, saliva contains various proteins, free amino acids, carbohydrates, urea, ammonia, creatinine, and mucin. Saliva is a complex biological medium and contains lipids, enzymes, hormones and mineral components - [100, 59, 81, 154].

The percentage of certain substances is determined by their plasma levels and the amount secreted. The percentage of lipids, glucose, and steroids in saliva is considerably less - [88] and potassium is five times greater than in blood. There is a high correlation between plasma and saliva in the content of androgens, aldosterone, cortisol, progesterone - [156].

Among a large number of components and indicators determined in saliva, electrolytes sodium and potassium are of special importance, as they are indirect indicators of the release of adaptive hormones and are most susceptible to the influence of stressogenic factors. Their content in salivary fluid changes in the course of professional activity more sharply than the concentration of other components [113, 97, 20, 42, 153, 197].

Currently, the sodium and potassium content of serum, urine, cerebrospinal fluid, and saliva are examined by many clinical diagnostic laboratories. Sodium is the main univalent cation in the extracellular fluid; potassium is the main intracellular cation.

It is advisable to determine the sodium content simultaneously with potassium. Sodium is involved in maintaining the constancy of the extracellular environment, it also has a number of regulatory effects. Thus, glucose transport into the cell depends on the presence of sodium in the intracellular medium: an increase in the intracellular concentration of sodium increases the entry of glucose into the cell. The maintenance of plasma sodium concentration within narrow limits is the result of the combined action of many regulatory systems. The hypothalamus, pituitary, epiphysis, adrenal glands, kidneys, and right atrial wall tissue are involved in the regulation. Increased sodium content in saliva is observed under heat and cold influences - [73, 177].

The study of the dynamics of sodium and potassium has a certain value and is considered as an indicator of increasing activity of the sympathoadrenal system, which has an inverse relationship with the indicators of trace elements in saliva. Heat and cold exposure and acute hypoxia has a significant effect on the content of sodium and potassium in biological fluids of the human body. The data on their dynamics allow us to obtain baseline information and make it possible to know the share of their participation in the mechanisms of adaptation formation to such extreme factors of impact on the organism as heat, cold, hypoxia and others [57, 73, 177].

The study of the potassium and sodium content of saliva in the altered gas environment allowed us to conclude that the potassium and sodium content in saliva is an informative indicator of the tension of regulatory mechanisms depending on the type features of the CNS - [97, 153].

Stability of potassium content in the organism is a consequence of balanced processes of its intake and excretion. The main reason for changes in the intracellular potassium content is a violation of the acid-base state. Potassium entering the body is distributed among body tissues within 24-30 hours. The entry of potassium into the cell through the plasma membrane is determined by many factors. Potassium channels provide passive permeability of the membrane for the cation. The movement of potassium is determined by the magnitude of the electrical potential and the concentration gradient. Potassium excretion results from a combination of filtration, reabsorption, and secretion processes. The Na/K transport system is involved in the process of potassium reabsorption. In adrenal cortex insufficiency, potassium excretion with urine decreases; at the same time, in adrenal cortex hyperactivity, increased sodium reabsorption leads to increased potassium excretion - [183]. Significant influence on the level of potassium in plasma is exerted by blood pH disturbance, as well as the content of anion HCO3- in blood, which reflects the degree of catabolic processes. Potassium excretion differs at different times of the day, which also affects the rhythm of glucocorticoid excretion - [82, 180, 186, 176].

The cells of the nervous system react quickly to the level of potassium in the plasma, which can explain the early appearance of neurological symptoms. The first signs of potassium deficiency are weakened reflexes, muscle hypotonia, weakness and asthenia. Hypokalemia is accompanied by abnormalities of conduction and rhythm of the heart, which is reflected in ECG changes on the ECG are also found at potassium concentrations above 6 mmol/L, that is, in hyperkalemia - [188]. It is established that hyperkalemia leads to impaired carbohydrate metabolism and causes changes in the content of cortisol in the blood - [181].

The interdependence of potassium depletion and impaired carbohydrate tolerance, as well as the decrease in plasma potassium in response to increased plasma catecholamine concentrations during stress is undisputed - [178].

At present, the methods for the determination of potassium content in biological fluids can be summarized as follows: flame photometry, ion-selective electrode potentiometry, flame atomic absorption spectrophotometry, and the use of crown ethers in colorimetric analysis - [176].

An important advantage of the combination of laboratory methods is that the degree of severity of the subjects' state of tension is characterized not by the absolute value of the increase or decrease of selected indicators, but by the dynamics of the relationship between them - [119, 59].

Ambrosioni E. et al. (1982) determined the content of twenty-one elements in saliva of healthy people by means of neutron activation and X-ray fluorescence analysis. They studied the dependence of saliva composition on sex, age, time of day and season of the year. The authors found clear circadian fluctuations in the content of sodium and potassium. They found that saliva composition was influenced only by time of day, while age, sex and season of the year had no significant effect. The revealed significant relationship of sodium and potassium concentrations with the time of day suggests the need to strictly regulate the time of saliva collection when studying the influence of other factors on its composition. At the same time, the optimal time for saliva collection is considered to be 10-11 am, because at this time the individual variability of saliva composition is the least pronounced - [148].

Changes in salivary glucose content during psychoemotional stress are of considerable interest. Data on the content of glucose in saliva are contradictory. A number of authors believe that in norm glucose does not penetrate from blood into saliva. At the same time, there is evidence that under stress the glucose content in saliva increases significantly. This duality of scientific data is probably due to the inadequacy of the methods used to determine glucose in studies by different authors [56, 42, 184, 151, 143].

Since the 90s, the glucose oxidase method has been widely used to determine glucose in biological fluids. The above-mentioned authors in their studies found a reliable increase in the amount of glucose in saliva during psychoemotional stress. At the same time, the increase in the glucose content in saliva during psychoemotional stress occurs under the influence of adrenaline, which increases glucose transport from blood to saliva [56, 143, 184, 151].

The increase in the amount of glucose in saliva under stress confirms the hypothesis about the dependence of the quantitative and qualitative composition of saliva on the functional state of the organism. Domestic and foreign researchers have revealed clear circadian fluctuations in glucose content. It was found that the circadian rhythm of glucose is stable and persists throughout life, as well as the revealed distinct circadian rhythm of noradrenaline and adrenaline levels in blood: maximum during the day and minimum during the night [21, 56].

Some authors emphasize the importance of glucose in those cases when the organism needs additional and rapidly increasing energy expenditure, for example, during emotional excitement, heavy muscular effort, in conditions causing a drop in body temperature - [58, 56, 132, 177, 143]. The important role of glucose in the body's energy is due to the rapidity of its oxidation, as well as the fact that it is quickly extracted from the depot and can be used in extreme situations for the body. In case of reduction of sugar in blood to 40 mg %, instead of the normal content of

100 mg % on average, sharp disorders of CNS activity are noted. Many researchers are convinced that the blood glucose content is influenced by the cerebral cortex. Proof of this is the increase in blood sugar and excretion of small amounts of it with urine in students, athletes in the pre-start period, when they are waiting for the signal to start the competition, the spectators of a soccer match and the substitute players who did not participate in the game, but worried about the success of their team.

The influence of the hypothalamus and cerebral cortex on glucose content is realized mainly through the sympathetic nervous system, which causes increased adrenaline secretion by the adrenal glands. Adrenaline also acts on the liver and muscles, causing glycogen mobilization. Thus, the action of adrenaline entails, firstly, the use of glycogen reserve of muscles as a source of energy for their work, and secondly, the increased flow of glucose from the liver into the blood, which can also be used by muscles in their work. They studied the functional state of the students' organism during the session. They noted an increase in glucose and potassium, and a decrease in sodium in saliva under the influence of nervous and emotional tension - [39, 143]. They also made an interesting observation that the changes in the above components of saliva were 2 times less in students of physical education faculty, who were constantly engaged in physical training.

Nicolcon N. [189] proposed to use the indicators of cortisol content in saliva as a convenient and reliable test to assess emotional stress. In case of insufficient secretion of glucocorticoids, which includes cortisol, the body's resistance to various harmful influences decreases. It has been noted that in pain, trauma, blood loss, overheating, hypothermia, and severe mental distress the secretion of glucocorticoids increases [74, 130, 158, 183]. This is explained by a reflex increase in adrenaline secretion by the cerebral layer of the adrenal glands. Adrenaline entering the bloodstream acts on the hypothalamus, causing the formation of corticoliberin, which promotes the formation of adrenocorticotropic hormone in the anterior lobe of the pituitary gland. This hormone is the factor that stimulates the production of glucocorticoids in the adrenal gland. Cortisol secretion has a diurnal character, with a minimum concentration in the late, evening and maximum in the early, morning hours, and the circadian rhythmicity of adrenal cortical hormones is independent of age and sex - [82, 188, 180, 186, 176, 183, 158].

Many authors describe in detail the mechanism of action of glucocorticosteroids, the main one being cortisol. In the cytoplasm of cells of different organs, there are receptor proteins capable of selectively attaching glucocorticosteroids. The hormone then enters the nucleus, interacts with chromatin and changes the rate of transcription of certain genes. Consequently, the amount of synthesis of the corresponding proteins also changes.

Currently, there are no universal tests that can provide an exhaustive answer to all questions of health assessment and functional state of the organism. Therefore, it is very important to choose the most informative methods of examination, taking into account their availability, compatibility, and the possibility of using them in vivo and during dynamic observations [41, 62, 57, 71, 174, 152].

Stress is based on nonspecific components. The most well-known and well-studied components of stress at present are activation of the sympathoadrenal system (SAS), release of liberins by the hypothalamus and further increase in the secretion of ACTH, thyroid and somatotropic hormones by the anterior lobe of the pituitary gland with subsequent peripheral adrenergic effects [27, 40, 43, 159].

It is quite obvious that at extreme magnitude of the stimulus or depletion of the reserve capabilities of the organism, stress can turn from a link of adaptogenesis into a link of pathogenesis - [94, 111] with characteristic phenomena of distress - [112] and the development of maladaptation - [95].

Combined exposure of the organism to various factors is characterized by a variety of responses determined by the spectrum of acting factors, their partial intensity and the state of individual resistance of the organism, i.e. functional state. Usually one has to observe the summation of the effects of activation of nonspecific defense mechanisms observed under each of the separately taken influences [103, 124].

The study of biochemical shifts (reactions) in response to ecopathogenic actions of factors will provide a more complete picture of the mechanisms of stability, development of adaptation reactions in the human body, to justify ways to optimize this process, to determine organizational, pedagogical and medical-social measures.

The principles of anticipatory cyto-biochemical screening during diagnostic and corrective measures to identify persons at risk of cardiovascular pathology (hypertensive type NDC, arterial hypertension) have now been substantiated. The essence of this principle consists in the primary indication of "sympathoadrenal status" based on the identification of the critical metabolic system. This allows to carry out reasonable measures for restorative correction and preventive therapy - [70, 103].

Among the biochemical mechanisms of adaptation under these conditions, an important role is attributed to the increase in the individual level of CAC activity and the tendency to increase the background (basal) values of blood pressure [86, 99, 63, 99, 76, 77, 187].

It is important to note that optimal adaptation processes are observed at moderate activation of CAS, and two-threefold excess of the background level of its activity is accompanied by the development of maladaptation disorders, which, in particular, in relation to the conditions of professional activity is manifested in a decrease in its quality by an increase in the number of erroneous actions - [105, 162, 166].

The results of long-term observations of individuals experiencing systematic psychoemotional loads associated with compensatory-adaptive changes in the organs and systems of the body indicate that these factors contribute to the development of hypertensive states and various morphofunctional regional and systemic disorders of the cardiovascular system (CVS) - [49, 52, 69, 64, 101, 101, 46, 61, 79, 145, 186, 169, 168, 168, 170].

It follows that the maintenance of the functional state of the organism in the optimal mode should be provided by the optimal level of CAC activity for a given individual, without exceeding the level followed by the failure of adaptation mechanisms of functional systems. To determine this level, a special criterion of individual control over the state of the mechanisms of the regulatory apparatus of the SAS itself was proposed [50, 77, 78]. A methodological approach to individual assessment of CAC activity using the indicator of β-adrenoreception of cell membranes (β-ARM) was developed, and its relationship with the severity of hypertensive states, as well as the reactions of the SSc to the performance of the information load test was determined [51, 52, 65, 66, 76, 53, 185, 163].

The index of β - adrenergic reactivity of erythrocyte membranes is an informative test to assess the dynamics of the functional state of the human organism, an integral indicator of its adaptation level and the probability of development of decompensated hyperadrenergic states, i.e. actually maladaptation processes.

The β-ARM indicator was determined by a method based on the use of peripheral blood erythrocytes as a model. It is known that to characterize the activity of CAS traditionally use quantitative assessment of secretion or excretion of catecholamines and their precursors, as well as the activity of enzymes of synthesis or deactivation of these substances in blood and tissues. Proceeding from the fact that the functional state of the CAC detector link - the adrenoreceptor apparatus of cell membranes - is under the control of feedback with the amount of adrenoactive substances acting on the cell, some researchers found it possible to use a quantitative index of cell membrane adrenoreception in relative units to determine CAC activity [89, 185, 163]. They developed and patented a method of β-ARM determination by the change in the functional state of erythrocytes in the presence of an adrenoactive substance [53, 116]. The unique role of the erythrocyte as a model living cell of the organism and the unique properties of its membranes can be judged by a number of works.

Thus, conformational changes in erythrocyte membranes under the action of biologically active substances, changes in the electron kinetic potential of erythrocytes were found, which indicates the mediated action of these substances on the permeability and ion transport in erythrocyte membranes. Biologically active substances, including adrenaline, change the electrical properties of the surface of red blood cells, significantly reducing the electrical charge of erythrocytes [22, 72].

In this process, a significant role is played by deformation of the membrane structure with a subsequent change in permeability to substances capable of neutralizing the surface electrical charge. BAS are not only adsorbed from cell membranes, but also interact with its components, causing conformational transformation in membrane proteins with subsequent changes in membrane permeability [121].

Currently, one of the methods that determine the individual status of the sympathoadrenal system is the study of membrane adrenoreactivity [22, 53, 72]. According to this method, β-adrenergic membrane reactivity (β-ARM) values in 90% of practically healthy people are in the range of 2.0 - 20.0 units. Individual values of β-ARM values are stable for many weeks and months under the condition of observance of the usual for a given person mode of labor and rest. At regular increase of CAC activity β-ARM values can increase up to 60 units. - [51, 116].

Thus, our analysis of the literature proves that at present there are practically no descriptions of comprehensive, adequate, non-invasive methods of examination of people living in regions with different ranks of anthropotechnogenic load. Consequently, the given general scientific data convince of the necessity of purposeful research on studying the content of sodium, potassium, glucose and cortisol in saliva as indicators of changes in the functional state of the human body in order to study the direction of adaptation reactions in migrants living in the conditions of the agro-industrial region with different ranks of anthropotechnogenic load, as well as for further use of the obtained results in mass examinations of various contingents of people non-invasively, All this served as a basis for the choice of the research topic.

2.1 Characteristics of the surveyed migrants living in the Lipetsk region with different ranks of anthropotechnogenic load

During the experiment, a test protocol was kept, which included questionnaire data, including surname, name, patronymic, home address, date of birth, gender, period of residence in regions with different ranks of anthropotechnogenic load.

The distribution of the examined persons by sex and age is presented in Fig. 1.

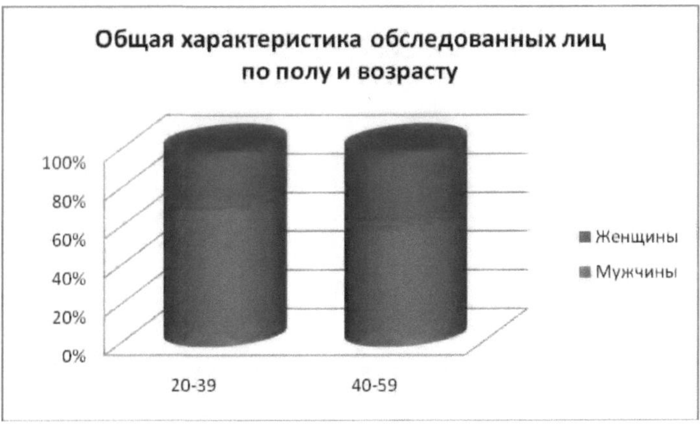

Fig. 1

The figure shows that 191 (55%) people were examined between the ages of 20-39 years and 156 (45%) were examined between the ages of 40-59 years. Among all those surveyed, 67% were men and 33% women.

The number of migrants living in the agro-industrial region with different ranks of anthropotechnogenic load is presented in Fig. 2.

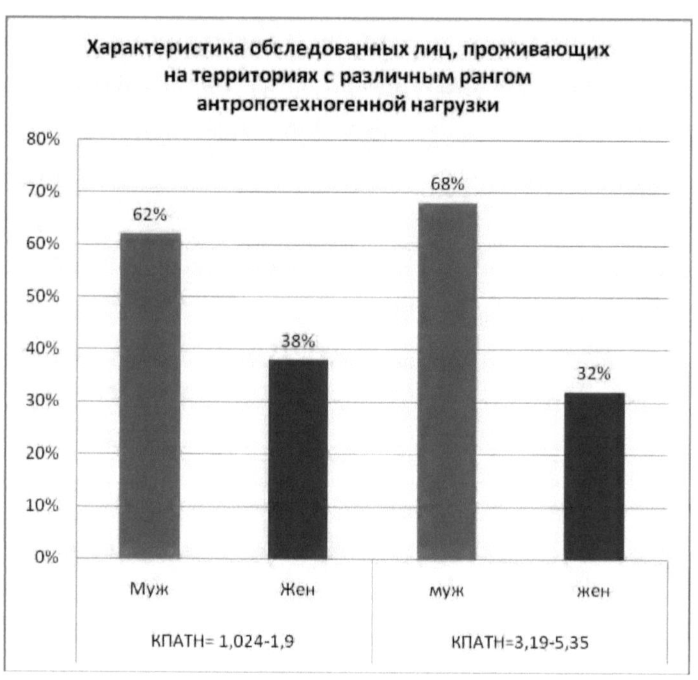

Fig. 2

The figure shows that in the area with low rank of anthropotechnogenic load 161 (46%) people were surveyed: men 106 (66%) and 55 (34%) women, and in the area with high rank of anthropotechnogenic load 186 (54%) people were surveyed: men 128 (69%) and 58 (31%) women.

Characterization of the Lipetsk region with a low rank of the quantitative indicator of anthropotechnogenic load (KPATN=1.024-1.9)

In the specific weight of eco-pathogenic environmental factors in the territories of Lipetsk region with a low level of anthropotechnogenic load prevailed: increased content of nitrates in drinking water over 3 MAC and increased level of gamma background over 5mSv. From the tentative list of environmental factors with their possible influence on the prevalence of some classes and groups of diseases in these areas, none of the most significant indicators for diseases of the genitourinary and endocrine systems was found to be present. These areas are considered safe according to the results of measurements of physical factors (noise, vibration, microclimate, EMF, illumination) at workplaces. Other environmental factors (physical, chemical) were registered at levels below the permissible values, which allowed ranking these territories of the region to refer them to areas with low rank of anthropotechnogenic load on the external environment (CPATN = 1.024 - 1.9).

Characterization of the Lipetsk region with a high rank of quantitative indicator of anthropotechnogenic load (CPATN=3.19-5.35)

The specific weight of ecopathogenic environmental factors in the territories of the Lipetsk region with a high level of anthropotechnogenic load prevailed: increased number of non-standard drinking water samples by chemical and microbiological indicators during 10 years of observation (4-17%), increased level of iron content in drinking water over 1 MAC, increased hardness of drinking water over 1 MAC, increased level of nitrates in drinking water over 1 MAC, the rank on the total indicator of drinking water is minimal (>5.39), growth of nitrogen oxides emissions into the atmosphere up to 270 th. tons and increased gamma background level of more than 5mSv. There was an increase in the volume of gross industrial waste of toxicity classes 1-4. According to the risk of atmospheric air impact on the health of urban population, the ecological and hygienic situation on the total atmospheric air pollution (criterion "P") was assessed as "strong" and "very strong", and for some chemical substances (dust, nitrogen dioxide, phenol, benzapyrene, formaldehyde, hydrogen sulfide, naphthalene, lead) concentrations exceeded MAC from 2 to 8 times, and they were priority in terms of hazard. The urban share of the contribution of chemical pollution of drinking water to the complex indicator was quite high and amounted to 33.5 %. At the same time, periodic increase of MPC of selenium, beryllium, arsenic, magnesium, cadmium, lead, iron was observed in the water of water intakes and water represented a high degree of potential danger for public health.

From the indicative list of environmental factors with their possible influence on the prevalence of certain classes and groups of diseases in these areas, none of the most significant indicators for diseases of the endocrine system was found to be present. These areas are unfavorable according to the results of measurements of physical factors (noise, vibration, microclimate, EMF, illumination) at women's workplaces. According to the CPATN criterion, the cities and districts of the area can be characterized as high-risk and high-risk zones with regard to diseases of the genitourinary system. A similar picture is observed in terms of ranking by the Pearson correlation coefficient of the total indicator of food quality and drinking water quality. The combination of exceeding the control levels for essentially significant indicators of environmental composition resulted in the ranking of these territories of the region by the complex indicator of anthropogenic load on the external environment to a high rank (CPATN=3.19-5.35)

2.2. Study of cardiovascular system, types of integral assessment of regulatory mechanisms of blood pressure and index of functional changes

In the course of the experiment, the cardiovascular system was assessed using such indicators as blood pressure (BP): systolic (SAD), diastolic (DBP), pulse pressure (PP), mean (Mean), minute (MOC) blood volume, cardiac index (CI) and specific peripheral vascular resistance (SPR), body area. IOC was determined by the formula: IOC = (1.43 x COC x HR + 2.53) / 1000 (l/min). SI was determined by the formula: SI = IOC/Stt (l/min/m$^{2)}$. Sr.D = (CAD - DAD) / 3 + DAD (mmHg). UPSS - according to the formula: UPSS = BPcr x80 / SI(din.s$^{-1.}$ see^{-5}).

On the basis of the listed indicators, the types of integral assessments of the regulatory mechanisms of blood pressure were determined.

An important condition of physiological examination is to take into account even small changes in the functional capabilities of the organism, which is essential for predicting unfavorable shifts and their prevention. In this case, it is necessary not only to analyze and process primary medical and physiological information, but also to obtain integral assessments based on objective statistically verified "weighting" of individual indicators. A number of functional indices well-proven in psychophysiological studies are used as such integral assessments, including the index of functional changes (IFI), the determination of which allows to objectively testify about the level of adaptation processes in the organism. The index of functional changes is calculated according to the formula: ИФИ=0,011хЧСС+0,014хСАД+0,008хДАД+0,014хВ+0,009хМТ-

0,009хР-0,27, где: HR - heart rate, beats/min; CAD - systolic blood pressure, mm Hg; DAD - diastolic blood pressure, mm Hg; B - age in years; MT - body weight in kg; P - height in cm. The conditional boundaries of the ranges of FTI values to distinguish different levels of adaptation are: satisfactory adaptation - up to 2.59; tension of adaptation mechanisms - from 2.60 to 3.09; unsatisfactory adaptation - from 3.09 to 3.49; failure of adaptation mechanisms - more than 3.50.

2.3.   Method for determining the concentration of sodium, potassium ions and Na/K ratio

To determine the concentration of sodium, potassium ions and Na/K ratio, saliva was collected by spitting into a test tube or by placing a cotton swab behind the cheek followed by centrifugation at 3000 - 20000 rpm for 5-30 minutes. To get rid of foam and viscosity of saliva due to mucin, a simple method of its denaturation - freezing and subsequent thawing of saliva - was used. For proper evaluation of the results, we took into account the conditions of collection - 1-3 hours after a meal. Collection was necessarily preceded by hygienic treatment of the mouth (rinsing), since dental plaque contains a lot of protein and enzymes. The standard method of sodium and potassium determination on biochemical ALKALI-microanalyzer type OR-266/I Radelix, Budapest, Hungary - the device is designed for fast and accurate determination of potassium and sodium ions concentration in biological fluids. One microvolume sample (volume not lower than 50 mm^3) is sufficient for measuring both parameters. The apparatus is practically suitable for the determination of potassium, sodium concentration of arbitrary solution. The registration was expressed in mmol/dm^3 .

2.4. Method for determination of glucose and cortisol concentration in saliva

Glucose concentration was determined by the glucose oxidase method. Modification of the glucose oxidase method of saliva examination consisted in determining the necessary amount of saliva and reagents, since the concentration of glucose in saliva is extremely small. It was found that the amount of saliva should be within 0.5 - 1 ml. The working solution was prepared according to the instructions. The standard glucose solution from the set is diluted twice: 2.3 ml of the solution and 7.2 ml of bidistilled water are mixed, 0.5 ml of the resulting mixture is taken, which is again diluted in 4.5 ml of water. The resulting glucose solution containing 100 μmol/L glucose is used as a standard solution. Determination is carried out according to the scheme presented in Table 3

Table 1

Determination of glucose concentration in saliva

Sample	Saliva (ml)	Deproteinism. p-r (ml)	Standard. p-r (ml)	Bidistil. water (ml)
Experienced	0.5	0.5	-	-
Standard		0.5	0.5	-
Idle		0.5	-	0.5

The contents of the samples are mixed, sedimented for 20 minutes and centrifuged at 3000 rpm for 20 minutes, 3 ml of the working solution is added to 0.5 ml of each sample.

The tubes are incubated in a thermostat at 37^0 C for 30 minutes and colorimetrically analyzed at 490 nm in a cuvette with a relative path length of 1cm against water.

Calculation: $\dfrac{\varepsilon_{on} - \varepsilon_{xon}}{\varepsilon_{cm} - \varepsilon_{xon}} \times 10 (ммоль/л)$

where ε - extinction of experimental, blank and standard samples, respectively (Dubova L.I., 1990).

Cortisol content in saliva was determined by radioimmunologic method using domestic kits Steron-T[125] - I and Steron-K -I-M.[125]

The study revealed that the content of hormones in saliva is significantly lower than in blood plasma, so we modified the method of their determination in saliva. After thawing, saliva was centrifuged at 4000 rpm for 10 min. For the study 1 ml of supernatant was taken. Due to the nonspecific "matrix" effect of saliva, apparently caused by mucin and other mucopolysaccharides, hormone extraction with diethyl ether was performed. In a test tube to 1ml of supernatant was added 5 ml of diethyl ether and shaken on a Vertex for 1 min, then the aqueous part was frozen. The ether was distilled off using a water-jet pump. For cortisol determination, the resulting dry residue was diluted with low molecular weight phosphate buffer to the original volume. 0.05 ml of the solution was taken for the study [88].

2.5. Method for determining the characterization of individual status of CAC-adrenergic responsiveness by changes in the functional state of erythrocytes

Control over the state of health of the subjects living in ecologically aggressive environment, as well as assessment of functional reserves and mechanisms of their provision, was carried out according to the indicator of beta-adrenergic reactivity of erythrocyte membranes. Activation of CAS is a stress-initiating factor that forms the danger of transition from the stage of stable adaptation to maladaptation. Identification of the initial stages of maladaptive processes can provide valuable material for preventing the consequences of adaptation failure. Unfavorable prognosis of changes in endurance and SSS functions can be associated with increased emotional reactivity and high hormonal activity in conditions of rest and physical activity. Activation of the sympathoadrenal (CAS) system belongs to one of the most well-studied stress-realizing factors that form the danger of transition from the stage of stable adaptation to dysadaptation, the emergence of destructive changes at the cellular level and dysregulatory changes at the systemic level.

Adrenoreactivity of the organism was evaluated by the effect of β-adrenoblocker on erythrocyte osmoresistance. For this purpose, 0.2 ml of peripheral blood was taken from a finger puncture with a glass pipette washed with anticoagulant. The blood sample in the presence of buffer solution was mixed with adrenergic reactive substance solution, incubated at room temperature for 15 min, then centrifuged for 10 min at 1500 rpm. The optical density of control and experimental samples against saline solution was measured at a wavelength of 540 nm using an electrophotocolorimeter KFK-2. The value of β-ARM was calculated according to the formula in conventional units. Normal values of β-ARM index are in the range from 2.0 to 20.0 units. At reduced adrenoreactivity the value of β-ARM exceeds 20.0 units.

2.6. Method of statistical processing of the research results.

An important stage of processing the collected experimental material is statistical (mathematical) processing of the research results. In our research we used methods of mathematical statistics. For these purposes, we chose study guides of various authors. The processed data were presented in tabular form, as well as in the form of graphical representation of the material. In the course of statistical processing of the study results, we made the determination of sample characteristics: arithmetic mean, dispersion (second central moment), unbiased estimation of dispersion, standard deviation, coefficient of variation. The laws of distribution of each parameter (concentration of sodium, potassium, glucose, cortisol, erythrocyte adrenoreactivity, cardiovascular system parameters) were also analyzed. On the basis of this analysis, histograms were constructed, on which we checked the normality of the law of distribution by means of such criteria as asymmetry and excess. Statistical processing of the obtained data was carried out on a computer using EXCEL program.

The methods used to examine the study population, the stages and scope of research are presented in Tables 2 and 3

Table 2

Methods used to survey the study population

Methods	Evaluated indicator
1- Determination of sodium and potassium concentration in saliva on biochemical ALKALI - microanalyzer of OR-266/I Radelix type (Menshikov V.V., 1987).	Concentration of sodium and potassium ions in saliva
2 Determination of glucose concentration in saliva using the glucose oxidase method (Dubova L.I. et al., 1990).	Glucose concentration in saliva
3 Determination of cortisol concentration in saliva by radioimmunologic method using domestic kits Steron-T^{125} -I and Steron-K^{125} I-M (Malov Y.S., Karpov V.A., 1994).	Cortisol concentration in saliva

4. study of the functional state of the cardiovascular system: heart rate, blood pressure by the Short method. Determination of functional change index	- heart rate (HR); - blood pressure (BP): systolic (CAD), diastolic (DBP), pulse pressure (PP), minute blood volume, total and specific peripheral vascular resistance, area of body mass, cardiac index. - types of integral assessments of the regulatory mechanisms of blood pressure - Identifying levels of adaptation
5. Determination of characterization of individual status of CAS-adrenoreactivity by the change in the functional state of erythrocytes in the presence of adrenoreactive substance using electrophotocolorimeter KFK-2 (Dlusskaya I.G., 1995).	- beta-adrenergic reactivity of erythrocyte membranes in conventional units using the beta-ARM reagent kit (AGAT-Med. Ltd., Moscow).

Table 3

Stages and scope of research

Stages	Study of social and medical peculiarities of the immigrant population of the region,	number surveyed	Number of studies

	evaluation of indicators of the study of the functional state of the organism and adaptive capabilities of the subjects.		
I	Analysis of the ecological zone of resident residence, labor in accordance with the level of CPATN, formation of observation groups	347	347
II	Survey of the region's immigrant population living in the territory with a low rank of anthropotechnogenic load.	161	2394
III	Survey of the region's immigrant population living in the territory with a high rank of anthropotechnogenic load.	186	2811
IV	Comparative and correlation analysis. Mathematical modeling of the adaptation process by regression analysis method based on the conducted comprehensive study.	347	3780
Total number of people examined and studies conducted		**347**	**9332**

Chapter 3. STATUS OF SYMPATOADRENAL SYSTEM LEVEL AND INDEX OF FUNCTIONAL CHANGES IN MIGRANT PERSONS LIVING IN REGIONS WITH DIFFERENT ANTHROPOTECHNOGENIC INJURIES

3.1 Basic hemodynamic parameters in migrant individuals with different lengths of residence in low and high rank anthropotechnogenic load conditions

The results of the study of SSS in men living in conditions with low rank of anthropotechnogenic load depending on age are reflected in Table 4

Table 4

Cardiovascular system indicators in men living in areas with low anthropotechnogenic load depending on age

Wo z pla nt	BP (mm.Hg.)			IOC	HR	SI	USP S
	DAD	GARD EN	Cf.				
20-39	69,9± 1,6	126,8±1, 7*	88,8±1,1* **	6,$\underline{15+0}$,1* **	65,5±3, 7*	3,$\underline{4+0}$, 1	24,1± 0,1
40-59	72,4±1, 09	134,3±1, 5	93,03 ± 1,7	6,$\underline{4+0}$,06	73,8±1, 6	3,$\underline{5+0}$, 09	25,0± 0,8

* p<0.001; **p<0.01; ***p<0.05

The table shows that in men aged 40-59 years under conditions with a low rank of anthropotechnogenic load insignificantly increase DAD, IOC and SI, UPSS practically does not change and significantly increase CAD, Cp and HR.

The results of the study of SSS in women living in conditions with low rank of anthropotechnogenic load depending on age are reflected in Table 5

Table 5

Cardiovascular system indicators in women living in areas with low anthropotechnogenic load depending on age

Wo z pla nt	BP (mm.Hg.)			IOC	HR	SI	USP S
	DAD	GARDE N	Cf.				
20-39	67,7±1,4*	129,2±1,05*	88,2±1,8*	6,3+0,08**	71,9±2,1**	3,5+0,14**	26,1 ± 0,1
40-59	80,2±1,9	139,4±2,03	99,9 ± 1,2	6,5+0,09	78,3±2,1	3,8+ 0,1	27,4 ± 1,3

* p<0.001; **p<0.01; ***p<0.05

The table shows that in women aged 40-59 years living in conditions with low rank of anthropotechnogenic load the indices of DA, CAD, Cp and HR increase significantly, IOC and SI increase insignificantly and UPSS practically does not change

The results of the study of SSS in men living in conditions with a high rank of anthropotechnogenic load depending on age are reflected in Table 6

Table 6

Cardiovascular system indicators in men living in areas with high anthropotechnogenic load depending on age

Age	BP (mm.Hg.)		Cf.	IOC	HR	SI	USPS
	DAD	GARDEN					
20-39	54,5 ± 2,1*	137,5 ± 4,2***	82,16 ± 1,3*	6,3+0,04***	84.3 ± 2.6***	3,8+0,01**	23,1 ± 0,8**
40-59	84,2 ± 5,2	143,8 ± 3,9	104,06 ± 2,2	6,5+0,15	76.3 ± 2.8	4,1 ± 0,12	26,7 ± 0,4

* p<0.001; **p<0.01; ***p<0.05

The table shows that in men aged 40-59 years living in conditions with a high rank of anthropotechnogenic load, there is a sharp increase in DAD (by 30.3 mm.Hg), which is associated with an increase in UPSS, there is also an increase in CAD, HR, Cp, and a slight increase in IOC and SI.

The results of SSS indices in women living in conditions with a high rank of anthropotechnogenic load depending on age are reflected in Table 7.

Table 7

Cardiovascular system indicators in women living in areas with high anthropotechnogenic load depending on age

Age	BP (mm.Hg.)			IOC	HR	SI	USPS
	DAD	GARDEN	Cf.				
20-39	66,1 ± 1,9*	128,5 ± 1,5*	86,9 ± 2,1*	6,4+0,09	69.7 ± 3.2***	3,9±0,07	27,5 ± 0,9
40-59	87,7 ± 2,02	149,1 ± 1,8	108,2 ± 1,9	6,5+0,01	74.2 ± 2.1	4,04 ± 0,08	28,4 ± 1,2

* p<0.001; **p<0.01; ***p<0.05

The table shows that in women aged 40-59 years under conditions with a high rank of anthropotechnogenic load, all studied indices, except for IOC and UPSS, are significantly increased.

The results of SSS indices in men aged 20-39 years living in conditions with low and high rank of anthropotechnogenic load are reflected in Fig.3

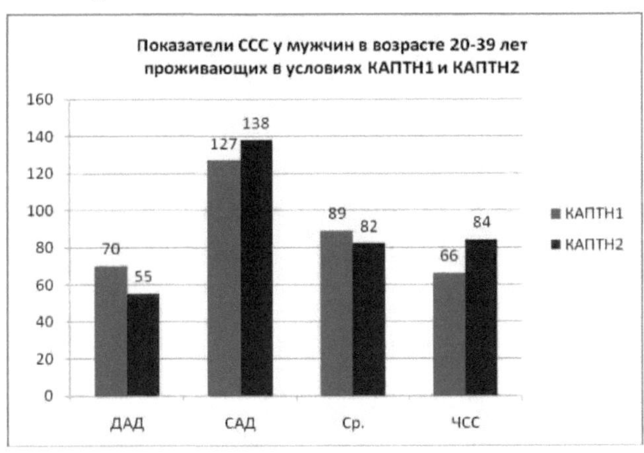

* p<0.001; **p<0.01; ***p<0.05 **Fig.3**

The figure shows that in men aged 20-39 years in conditions with a high rank of anthropotechnogenic load, there is a significant decrease in SAD and HR, which is associated with a slight decrease in PSS. There is a significant increase in SAD and HR. The results of SSS indices in men aged 40-59 years living in conditions with low and high rank of anthropotechnogenic load are reflected in Fig. 4

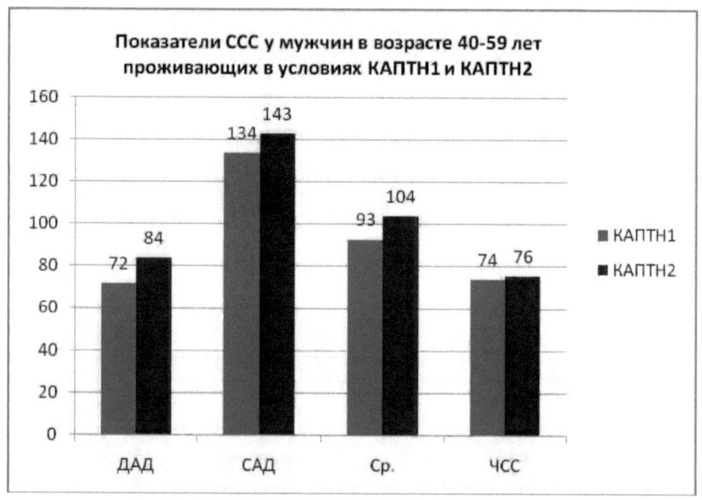

Fig. 4

The figure shows that in men aged 40-59 years in conditions with a high rank of anthropotechnogenic load all the studied indicators increase. It is noteworthy that in conditions with a high rank of anthropotechnogenic load, in men aged 20-39 years, DAD significantly decreases, and in men aged 40-59 years, this indicator significantly increases.

The results of SSS indices in women aged 20-39 years living in conditions with low and high rank of anthropotechnogenic load are reflected in Fig. 5

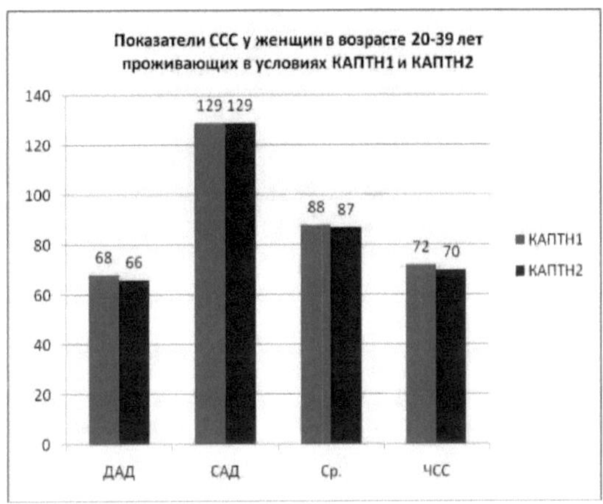

Fig. 6

The figure shows that in women aged 20-39 years in conditions with high rank of anthropotechnogenic load, all indicators are almost the same as in conditions with low rank of anthropotechnogenic load.

The results of SSS indices in women aged 40-59 years living in conditions with low and high rank of anthropotechnogenic load are reflected in Fig. 7

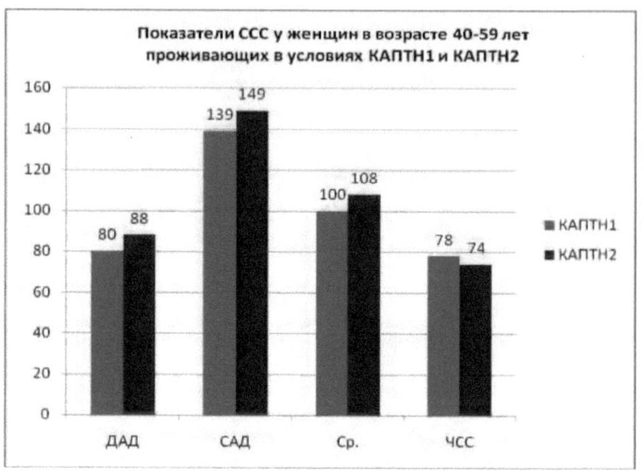

Fig. 7

The figure shows that in women aged 40-59 years in conditions with a high rank of anthropotechnogenic load, all indices, except IOC, increase.

The results of SSS indices in men and women aged 20-39 years living in conditions with a low rank of anthropotechnogenic load are reflected in Table 8

The table shows that SSS indices in men aged 20-39 years living in conditions with a low rank of anthropotechnogenic load practically do not differ from those in women.

Table 8

Cardiovascular system indices in men and women living in areas with low rank of anthropotechnogenic load at the age of 20-39 years old

Paul	BP (mm.Hg.)						
	DAD	GARDEN	Cf.	IOC	HR	SI	USPS

| Husb and ranks | 69,9± 1,6 | 126,8±1,7 | 88,86 ± 1,1 | 6,15+0,1 | 65,5±3,7*** | 3,4+0,1 | 24,1 ± 0,1*** |
| Wife wom en | 67,7±1,4 | 129,2±1,05 | 88,2 ± 1,8 | 6,3+0,08 | 71,9±2,1 | 3,5+0,14 | 26,1 ± 0,1 |

***p<0,05

The results of SSS indices in men and women aged 40-59 years living in conditions with a low rank of anthropotechnogenic load are reflected in Table 9

Table 9

Cardiovascular indices in men and women living in areas with low rank of anthropotechnogenic load at the age of 40-59 years old

Paul	BP (mm.Hg.)						
	DAD	GARDE N	Cf.	IOC	HR	SI	USP S
Husb and ranks	72,4±1,0 9**	134,3±1, 5***	93,0 3 ± 2,7* **	6,4+0 ,06	73,8±1,6 ***	3,5+0 ,09	25,0 ± 0,8
Wom en Ny	80,2±1,9	139,4±2, 03	99,9 ± 3,2	6,5+0 ,09	78,3±2,1	3,8+ 0,1	27,4 ± 1,3

**p<0.01; ***p<0.05

The table shows that all indices of SSS in women aged 40-59 years living in conditions with low rank of anthropotechnogenic load are increased in relation to those in men.

The results of SSS indices in men and women aged 20-39 years living in conditions with a high rank of anthropotechnogenic load are reflected in Table 10

table 10

Cardiovascular indices in men and women living in areas with high anthropotechnogenic load at the age of 20-39 years old

Paul	BP (mm.Hg.)			IOC	HR	SI	USPS
	DAD	GAR DEN	Cf.				
Men	54,5 ± 2,1*	137,5 ± 2,2**	82,16 ± 1,3**	6,3+0,04	84.3 ± 2.6**	3,8+ 0,01	23,1 ± 0,8
Women	66,1 ± 1,9	128,5 ± 1,5	88,9 ± 2,1	6,4+0,09	69.7 ± 3.2	3,9 ± 0,07	27,5 ± 0,9**

* p<0.001; **p<0.01;

The table shows that in women aged 20-39 years living in conditions with high rank of anthropotechnogenic load, there is a significant increase in MAP, which can be explained by an increase in PPSS. They also have an increase in Cp, and CAD and HR decrease. MOC and SI in women practically do not differ from those in men.

The results of SSS indices in men and women aged 40-59 years living in conditions with a high rank of anthropotechnogenic load are reflected in Table 11

Cardiovascular system indices in men and women living in areas with high anthropotechnogenic load at the age of 40-59 years old

Paul	BP (mm.Hg.)			IOC	HR	SI	USPS
	DAD	GAR DEN	Cf.				
Men	84,2 ± 5,2	143,8 ± 3,9***	104,1 ± 2,2***	6,5+0,1 5	76.3 ± 2.8	4,1 ± 0,12	26,7 ± 0,4***
Women	87,7 ± 2,02	149,1 ± 1,8	108,2 ± 1,9	6,5+0,0 1	74.2 ± 2.1	4,04 ± 0,08	28,4 ± 1,2

***p<0,05

The table shows that in women aged 40-59 years living in conditions with a high anthropotechnogenic load rank, MAP, CAD, SR. and CRP increase compared to the data of men. MOC, SI and HR practically do not differ from those in men.

Thus, a comparative analysis of age-specific parameters of the SSS shows that in men aged 40-59 years under conditions with low anthropotechnogenic load rank, DA, MOC and SI increase insignificantly and CAD, Cp and HR increase significantly. Similar changes are observed in women, but with a more significant increase in SAD. In conditions with a high rank of anthropotechnogenic load in men, there is a sharp increase in DA (by 30.3 mmHg), which is associated with an increase in UPSS, there is also an increase in CAD, HR, CBC and a slight increase in IOC and SI. In women, to a lesser extent, there is an increase in MAP, as they have practically no change in ROS.

The comparative analysis of SSS indices depending on the severity of ecopathogenic factors shows that in men aged 20-39 years in conditions with a high rank of anthropotechnogenic load, there is a significant decrease in SAD and HR, which is associated with some decrease in EPSS. There is a significant increase in SAD and HR, and at the age of 40-59 all studied parameters increase. It is noteworthy that in conditions with a high rank of anthropotechnogenic load in men at the age of 20-39 years DAD significantly decreases, and at the age of 40-59 years this indicator significantly increases. In women aged 20-39 years in conditions with a high rank of anthropotechnogenic load all indices practically remain the same as in conditions with a low rank of anthropotechnogenic load, and at the age of 40-59 years all indices, except IOC, increase.

The comparative analysis of SSS in men and women shows that in men aged 20-39 years, living in conditions with low rank of anthropotechnogenic load, the studied indices practically do not differ from those in women, and at the age of 40-59 years, all indices are smaller. In conditions with a high rank of anthropotechnogenic load in women at the age of 20-39 years significantly increases DAD, Cp, and CAD and HR decrease, IOC and SI practically do not differ from those in men. At the age of 40-59 years, DAD, CAD, SR. and HR increase, and IOC, SI and HR practically do not differ from those in men.

The index of functional changes (FFI) was used for quantitative assessment of adaptive capabilities. It was found that the adaptive capabilities of the organism depend on the period of residence in new conditions. The results of the distribution of migrants depending on the period of residence with regard to the level of adaptation are shown in Fig. 8

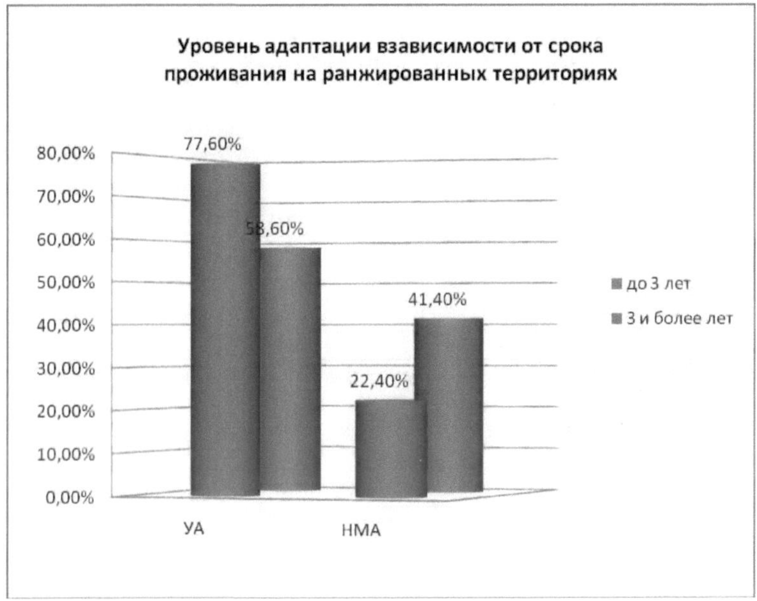

Fig. 8

The figure shows that among those surveyed with the period of residence up to 3 years, 77.6% are persons with satisfactory adaptation (SA) and 22.4% - with strained adaptation mechanisms (NMA). Among those surveyed with a period of residence of 3 years and more, the number of persons with AA decreases to 58.6%, and the number of persons with NMA increases twofold (41.4%)

3.2.   Evaluation of integral clinical assessments of regulatory

Blood pressure mechanisms in migrant individuals with different duration of residence in low and high rank anthropotechnogenic load conditions

The prevalence of types of regulatory mechanisms of blood pressure in men depending on age, living in conditions with low rank of anthropotechnogenic load is reflected in Table 12.

Table 12

Types of BP regulatory mechanisms (%) in age-dependent men living in areas with low anthropotechnogenic load ranking

Age	Integral assessment (functional diagnosis) - status			
	Normotoni penal	Borderline conditions	Hypotony penal	Hypertensio n penal
20-39 years old	14,2	11,7	5	69,1
40-59 years old	13,9	14,6	3,1	68,4

The table shows that in conditions with a low rank of anthropotechnogenic load, most of the examined men (69.1%) at the age of 20-39 years have a hypertensive type of BP regulatory mechanism. Only every seventh of the examined men has the normotonic type. The same pattern is observed among the examined men aged 40-59 years.

The prevalence of types of regulatory mechanisms of blood pressure in women depending on age living in conditions with low anthropotechnogenic load is shown in Table 13.

Table 13

Types of BP regulatory mechanisms (%) in age-dependent women living in areas with low anthropotechnogenic load ranking

Age	Integral assessment (functional diagnosis) - status			
	Normotoni penal	Borderline conditions	Hypotony penal	Hypertensio n penal
20-39 years old	9,1	15,9	4,5	70,5
40-59 years old	4,7	17,9	6,5	70,9

The table shows that in conditions with a low rank of anthropotechnogenic load, the majority of the examined women (70%) at the age of 20-39 and 40-59 years have a hypertonic type of BP regulatory mechanism. In women aged 40-59 years the number of persons with normotonic type decreases twice.

The prevalence of types of regulatory mechanisms of blood pressure in men depending on age living in conditions with high anthropotechnogenic load is shown in Table 14.

Table 14

Types of BP regulatory mechanisms (%) in men depending on age living in areas with high anthropotechnogenic load ranking

Age	Integral assessment (functional diagnosis) - status			
	Normotoni penal	Borderline conditions	Hypotony penal	Hypertension penal
20-39 years old	7,1	11,8	0	81,1
40-59 years old	8,6	13,1	0	78,3

The table shows that in conditions with a high rank of anthropotechnogenic load, the majority of examined men aged 20-39 (81.1%) and 40-59 (78.3%) years have a hypertensive type of BP regulatory mechanism. In both age groups there are no persons with hypotonic type.

The prevalence of types of regulatory mechanisms of blood pressure in women depending on age living in conditions with high anthropotechnogenic load is shown in Table 15.

Table 15

Integral clinical assessment of BP regulatory mechanisms (%) in women depending on age living in areas with high anthropotechnogenic burden

Age	Integral assessment (functional diagnosis) - status			
	Normotoni penal	Borderline conditions	Hypotony penal	Hypertension penal
20-39 years old	7,4	16,6	0	76,0
40-59 years old	12,3	7,3	0	79,1

The table shows that in conditions with a high rank of anthropotechnogenic load, most of the examined women aged 20-39 (76%) and 40-59 (79.1%) years have a hypertensive type of BP regulatory mechanism. In both age groups there are no persons with hypotonic type. At the age of 40-59 years, the number of examined women with normotonic type increases and the number of persons with borderline condition decreases twice.

The prevalence of types of regulatory mechanisms of blood pressure in men aged 20-39 years, living in conditions with low and high rank of anthropotechnogenic load is reflected in Fig. 9

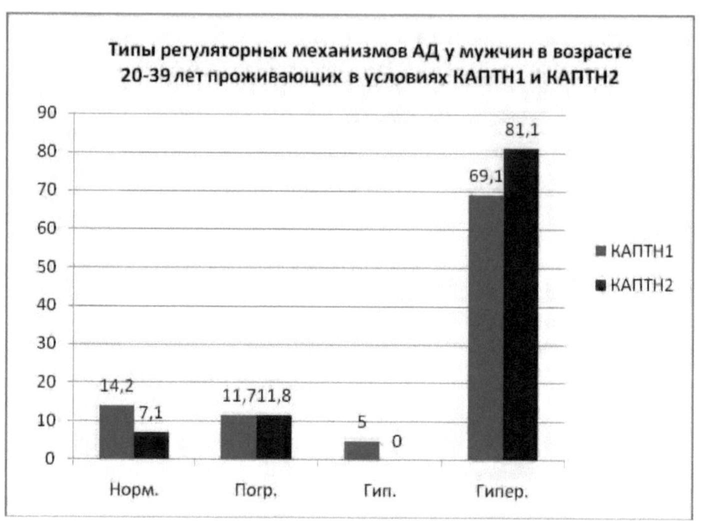

Fig. 9

The figure shows that in men aged 20-39 years in conditions with a high rank of anthropotechnogenic load, the number of persons with normotonic type decreases twice, there are no persons with hypotonic type and the number of persons with hypertensive type increases by 12%.

The prevalence of types of regulatory mechanisms of blood pressure in men aged 40-59 years living in conditions with low and high rank of anthropotechnogenic load is shown in Fig. 10

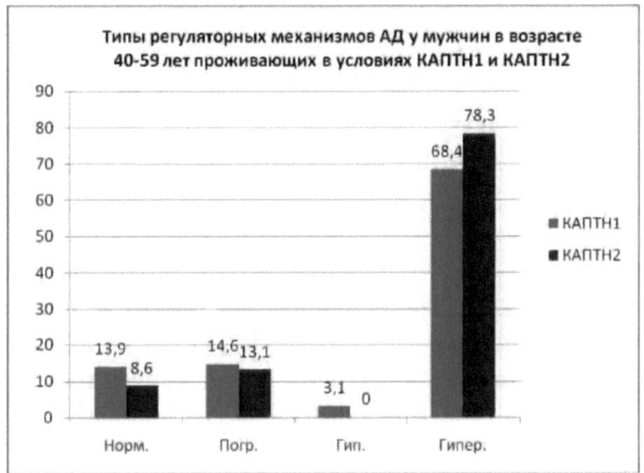

Fig. 10

The figure shows that the dynamics of types of BP regulatory mechanisms in men aged 40-59 years in conditions with high rank of anthropotechnogenic load is the same as in the age of 20-39 years.

The prevalence of types of regulatory mechanisms of blood pressure in women aged 20-39 years, living in conditions with low and high rank of anthropotechnogenic load is shown in Fig. 11

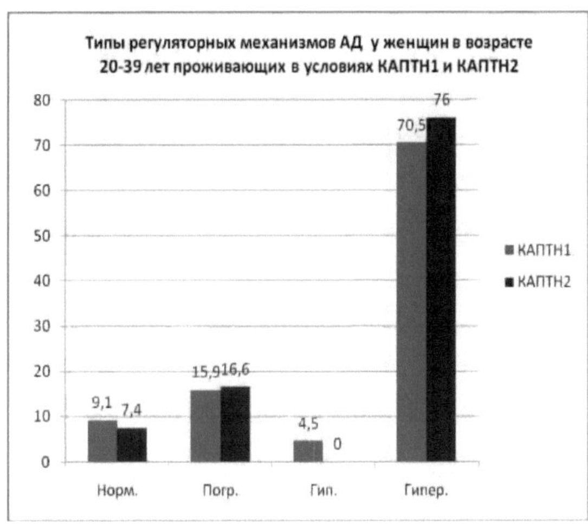

Fig. 11

The figure shows that in women aged 20-39 years in conditions with high rank of anthropotechnogenic load there are no individuals with hypotonic type and the number of individuals with hypertensive type increases.

The prevalence of types of regulatory mechanisms of blood pressure in women aged 40-59 years living in conditions with low and high rank of anthropotechnogenic load is shown in Fig. 12

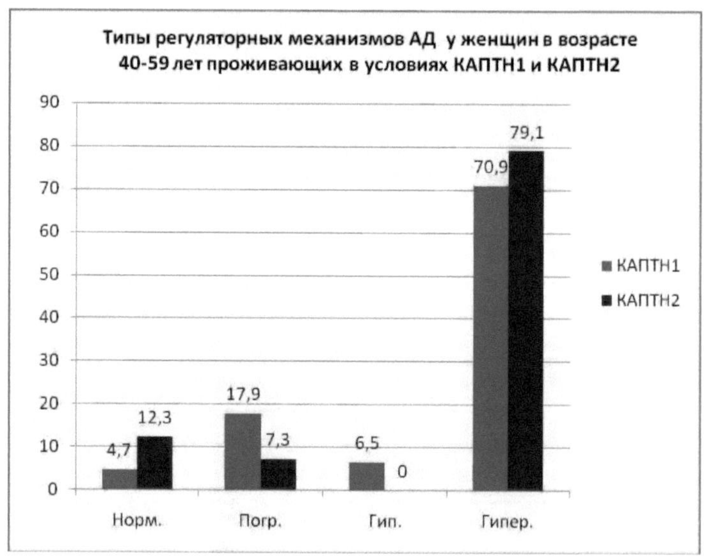

Fig. 12

The figure shows that in women aged 40-59 years in conditions with a high rank of anthropotechnogenic load in three times the number of persons with normotonic type increases, in more than two times the number of those examined with borderline condition decreases, there are no persons with hypotonic type and almost by 10% the number of persons with hypertensive type increases.

The prevalence of types of regulatory mechanisms of blood pressure in men and women aged 20-39 years living in conditions with a low rank of anthropotechnogenic load is shown in Table 16.

Table 16

Types of BP regulatory mechanisms (%) in men and women aged 20-39 living in areas with low anthropotechnogenic load ranking

Paul	Integral assessment (functional diagnosis) - status			
	Normotoni penal	Borderline conditions	hypotensio n penal	Hypertensi on penal
Men	14,2	11,7	5	69,1
Women	9,1	15,9	4,5	70,5

The table shows that the number of persons with normotonic type decreases and the number of persons with borderline state increases among the examined women aged 20-39 years in conditions with low rank of anthropotechnogenic load in comparison with the examined men.

The prevalence of types of regulatory mechanisms of blood pressure in men and women aged 40-59 years, living in conditions with low rank of anthropotechnogenic load is reflected in Table 17.

The table shows that among the examined women aged 40-59 years in conditions with low rank of anthropotechnogenic load in comparison with the examined men the number of persons with normotonic type decreases three times and the number of persons with hypotonic type increases two times.

Table 17

Types of BP regulatory mechanisms (%) in men and women aged 40-59 years living in areas with low anthropotechnogenic load ranking

Paul	Integral assessment (functional diagnosis) - status			
	Normotoni penal	Borderline conditions	hypotensio n penal	Hypertensi on penal
Men	13,9	14,6	3,1	68,4
Women	4,7	17,9	6,5	70,9

The prevalence of types of regulatory mechanisms of blood pressure in men and women aged 20-39 years living in conditions with a high rank of anthropotechnogenic load is reflected in Table 18.

Table 18

Types of BP regulatory mechanisms (%) in men and women aged 20-39 years living in areas with high anthropotechnogenic load ranking

Paul	Integral assessment (functional diagnosis) - status

	Normotoni penal	Borderline conditions	hypotension penal	Hypertension penal
Men	7,1	11,8	0	81,1
Women	7,4	16,6	0	76,0

The table shows that among the examined women aged 20-39 years in conditions with a high rank of anthropotechnogenic load in comparison with the examined men the number of persons with borderline condition increases and decreases with hypertonic type. Among the examined men and women there are no persons with hypotonic type.

The prevalence of types of regulatory mechanisms of blood pressure in men and women aged 40-59 years living in conditions with high anthropotechnogenic load is shown in Table 19.

Table 19

Integral clinical assessment of BP regulatory mechanisms (%) in men and women aged 40-59 years living in areas with high anthropotechnogenic load ranking

Paul	Integral assessment (functional diagnosis) - status			
	Normotoni penal	Borderline conditions	hypotension penal	Hypertension penal
Men	8,6	13,1	0	78,3
Women	12,3	7,3	0	79,1

The table shows that among the examined women aged 40-59 years in conditions with a high rank of anthropotechnogenic load in comparison with the examined men, the number of persons with normotonic type increases and the number of persons with borderline condition decreases almost twice. Among the examined men and women there are no persons with hypotonic type.

Thus, in conditions with a low rank of anthropotechnogenic load, the majority of the examined women (70%) at the age of 20-39 and 40-59 years have a hypertensive type of BP regulatory mechanism. In conditions with high anthropotechnogenic load rank the number of examined women with hypertensive type increases up to 79.1% and there are no persons with hypotonic type. Among the examined men in conditions with a high rank of anthropotechnogenic load the number of persons with normotonic type decreases twice, there are no persons with hypotonic type and the number of persons with hypertensive type increases by 12%. It was noted that among the examined women aged 40-59 years in conditions with low rank of anthropotechnogenic load in comparison with the examined men the number of persons with normotonic type decreases three times and the number of persons with hypotonic type increases two times.

The results of the types of BP regulatory mechanisms in men depending on the period of their residence in conditions with low anthropotechnogenic load are reflected in Table 20

Table 20

Types of BP regulatory mechanisms in men depending on the period of residence in low-rank anthropotechnogenic conditions

Length of stay	Types of BP regulatory mechanisms		

	Normotoni penal	borderline conditions	hypotensio n penal	Hypertensi on penal
Up to 3 years	7,0	11,5	3,2	78,3
3 or more	14,2	8,9	0	76,9

The table shows that in conditions with low rank of anthropotechnogenic load the number of examined men with hypertensive type practically does not change depending on the period of residence. With increasing duration of residence in the ranked territories there is an increase in the number of persons with normotonic type, a decrease in the number of persons with borderline condition and no persons with hypotonic type.

The results of the types of BP regulatory mechanisms in women depending on the period of their residence in conditions with a low rank of anthropotechnogenic load are reflected in Table 21

Table 21

Types of BP regulatory mechanisms in women depending on the period of residence in low-rank anthropotechnogenic conditions

Length of stay	Types of AD regulatory mechanisms			
	Normotoni penal	borderline conditions	Hypotony penal	Hypertensi on penal
Up to 3 years	10,2	12,9	3,1	73,8
3 or more	20,1	6	0	73,9

The table shows that in conditions with a low rank of anthropotechnogenic load the number of examined women with hypertensive type practically does not change depending on the period of residence. With increasing duration of residence in the ranked territories, there is an increase in the number of persons with normotonic type, a decrease in the number of persons with borderline condition and no persons with hypotonic type.

The results of the types of BP regulatory mechanisms in men depending on the period of their residence in conditions with high anthropotechnogenic load are reflected in Table 22

Table 22

Types of BP regulatory mechanisms in men depending on the period of residence in conditions with high anthropotechnogenic load ranking

Length of stay	Types of BP regulatory mechanisms			
	Normotoni penal	borderline conditions	hypotensio n penal	Hypertensi on penal
Up to 3 years	3,8	14,3	0	81,9
3 or more	13,6	7,5	0	78,9

The table shows that in conditions with a high rank of anthropotechnogenic load the number of examined men with hypertensive type practically does not change depending on the period of residence. With increasing duration of residence in the ranked territories the number of persons with normotonic type increases 4 times, the number of persons with borderline condition decreases two times and there are no persons with hypotonic type.

The results of the types of BP regulatory mechanisms in women depending on the period of their residence in conditions with high anthropotechnogenic load are reflected in Table 23

Table 23

Types of BP regulatory mechanisms in women depending on the period of residence in conditions with high anthropotechnogenic load ranking

Length of stay	Types of BP regulatory mechanisms			
	Normotoni penal	borderline conditions	hypotensio n penal	Hypertensi on penal
Up to 3 years	9,0	13,7	0	77,3
3 or more	18,2	7,5	0	74,3

The table shows that in conditions with a high rank of anthropotechnogenic load the number of examined women with hypertensive type practically does not change depending on the period of residence. With increasing duration of residence in the ranked territories, the number of persons with normotonic type increases twice, the number of persons with borderline condition decreases twice, and there are no persons with hypotonic type.

The results of the types of BP regulatory mechanisms in men and women with the period of residence up to three years in conditions with a low rank of anthropotechnogenic load are reflected in Table 24.

Table 24

Types of BP regulatory mechanisms in men and women with up to 3 years of residence in conditions with low rank of anthropotechnogenic load

Paul	Types of BP regulatory mechanisms			
	Normotoni penal	borderline conditions	hypotension penal	Hypertension penal
Men	7,0	11,5	3,2	78,3
Women	10,2	12,9	3,1	73,8

The table shows that the number of persons with normotonic type increases and the number of persons with hypertensive type decreases in the examined women with the period of residence up to three years in conditions with low rank of anthropotechnogenic load in comparison with the examined men.

The results of the types of BP regulatory mechanisms in men and women with 3 and more years of residence in conditions with low rank of anthropotechnogenic load are reflected in Table 25

Table 25

Types of BP regulatory mechanisms in men and women with 3 and more years of age in conditions with low rank of anthropotechnogenic load

Paul	Types of BP regulatory mechanisms			
	Normotoni penal	borderline conditions	hypotensio n penal	Hypertensi on penal
Men	14,2	8,9	0	76,9
Women	20,1	6	0	73,9

The table shows that the number of persons with normotonic type increases and the number of persons with hypertensive type decreases in the examined women with the period of residence of 3 and more years in conditions with low rank of anthropotechnogenic load in comparison with the examined men.

The results of the types of BP regulatory mechanisms in men and women with the period of residence up to 3 years in conditions with a high rank of anthropotechnogenic load are reflected in Table 26

Table 26

Types of BP regulatory mechanisms in men and women with up to 3 years of age in conditions with a high rank of anthropotechnogenic load

Paul	Types of BP regulatory mechanisms			
	Normotoni penal	borderline conditions	hypotensio n penal	Hypertensi on penal
Men	3,8	14,3	0	81,9

| Women | 9,0 | 13,7 | 0 | 77,3 |

The table shows that the number of persons with normotonic type increases three times in the examined women with the period of residence up to 3 years in conditions with a high rank of anthropotechnogenic load in comparison with the examined men and decreases with hypertonic type.

The results of the types of BP regulatory mechanisms in men and women with 3 and more years of residence in conditions with high anthropotechnogenic load are reflected in Table 27

Table 27

Types of BP regulatory mechanisms in men and women with 3 or more years of age in conditions with a high rank of anthropotechnogenic load

Paul	Types of BP regulatory mechanisms			
	Normotoni penal	borderline conditions	Hypotony penal	Hypertensio n penal
Men	13,6	7,5	0	78,9
Women	18,2	7,5	0	74,3

The table shows that the number of persons with normotonic type increases and the number of persons with hypertensive type decreases in the examined women with the period of residence of 3 and more years in conditions with high rank of anthropotechnogenic load in comparison with the examined men.

Thus, among men and women who lived in conditions with low and high rank of anthropotechnogenic load up to 3 years and more, the same number of persons with hypertensive type of BP regulatory mechanisms is observed. With increasing duration of residence in the ranked territories among men and women there is an increase in the number of persons with normotonic type, a decrease with borderline state and no persons with hypotonic type.

It was noted that in conditions with low and high rank of anthropotechnogenic load in the examined women with the period of residence up to three years and more compared to the examined men, the number of persons with normotonic type increases and the number of persons with hypertonic type decreases.

3.3 Beta-adrenergic reactivity of erythrocyte membranes in migrants living in low and high rank anthropotechnogenic load conditions

The analysis of erythrocyte membrane beta-adrenergic reactivity (β-ARM) in migrants living in different conditions of anthropogenic load shows that the β-ARM indicator underwent a number of changes that depended on the sex and age of the subjects.

The results of the studies presented in Table 28

Table 28

β-ARM in subjects living in territories with low anthropotechnogenic load ranking

On the contrary	β-adrenergic responsiveness of erythrocyte membranes (in U.S. dollars)

	Men (n=106)	Women (n=55)
20-39	24,5±1,7	22,1±0,9
40-59	22,6±2,3	20,3±2,3

As can be seen from the table, in men of the first age group of subjects, the β-ARM index exceeded the physiological norm by 22.5% and by 9.5% of the same index in older men. Comparison of the obtained results statistically reliably indicates that with age the adaptation processes in migrant individuals proceed with less pronounced tension of regulatory mechanisms. When the activity of CAC increases, protective desensitization of cell membranes develops, which leads to an increase in β-ARM indices in blood. The increase in CAC activity in men of different age groups serves as one of the manifestations of deep adaptation restructuring of the organism as a result of prolonged action of social, industrial and environmental stress factors.

Other indicators were obtained in the study of migrant women. In the examined women of the first age group, the β-ARM indicator slightly (10.5%) exceeded the upper limit of the physiological norm, and in older women it was within the established physiological norm.

The analysis of the obtained results allows us to conclude that the state of the organism of the examined women living in areas with a low rank of anthropogenic load is characterized by satisfactory adaptation to environmental conditions and they have sufficient functional reserves to maintain homeostasis with minimal stress of regulatory systems.

The study of CAC activity according to the β-ARM indicator in migrants living in aggressive environmental conditions, i.e. in areas with a high rank of anthropotechnogenic load, showed that the action of unfavorable environmental factors leads to significant disorders within and between the functional systems of the body.

The results of the research are presented in Table 29

As can be seen from the table, the β-ARM index in women was low compared to the norm and tended to decrease to normal values with increasing age. The data indicate signs of adaptive restructuring in the life-supporting systems of their organism and emphasize the resistance of the organism to eco-pathogenic environmental factors.

Table 29

β-ARM in subjects living in territories with a high rank of anthropotechnogenic load

On the contrary	β-adrenergic responsiveness of erythrocyte membranes (in U.S. dollars)	
	Men (n=128)	Women (n=58)
20-39	34,6±2,05***	23,4±1,1***
40-59	29,8±1,3	21,1±1,2

***p<0,05

In young men living in areas with a high rank of anthropotechnogenic load, the β-ARM index is 1.7 times higher than the norm and decreases by 15% in the blood of older migrant men.

Increased ß-ARM values in all examined men indicate a decrease in their adrenoreactivity at the cellular and systemic levels, which is a manifestation of a nonspecific defense mechanism against the destructive effect of increased catecholamines in conditions of prolonged psychoemotional and ecopathogenic stress. This indicates a change in the processes of synthesis, deposition and metabolism of catecholamines, as well as in the sensitivity (desensitization) of the receptor apparatus of erythrocyte cell membranes; this is especially revealed in young people. These changes can be considered as an unfavorable prognostic criterion for the risk of diseases, in the pathogenesis of which the leading role is attributed to the activity of CAC.

The obtained data are in direct correlation with changes in physiological indicators of the intensity of adaptation processes in the examined male migrants. In case of mobilization of protective mechanisms of adaptation in male migrants and intensive exposure to eco-pathogenic environmental factors, as well as psychoemotional stress associated with the change of place of residence and specificity of organism functioning in new conditions, the protective and modulating function of desensitization may be predominant, and this will be manifested in them at the systemic level by a more pronounced stress of physiological parameters. This will undoubtedly lead to decompensated hyperadrenergic states and development of SS pathology.

Chapter 4. changes in the biochemical composition of saliva in migrant persons living in regions with different anthropotoxic loadings

4.1. Changes in the electrolyte composition of saliva (sodium, potassium ion concentrations and Na/K ratio)

The results of changes in sodium, potassium, Na/K ratio in saliva of men living in areas with low and high rank of anthropotechnogenic load in comparison with background are reflected in Fig. 13

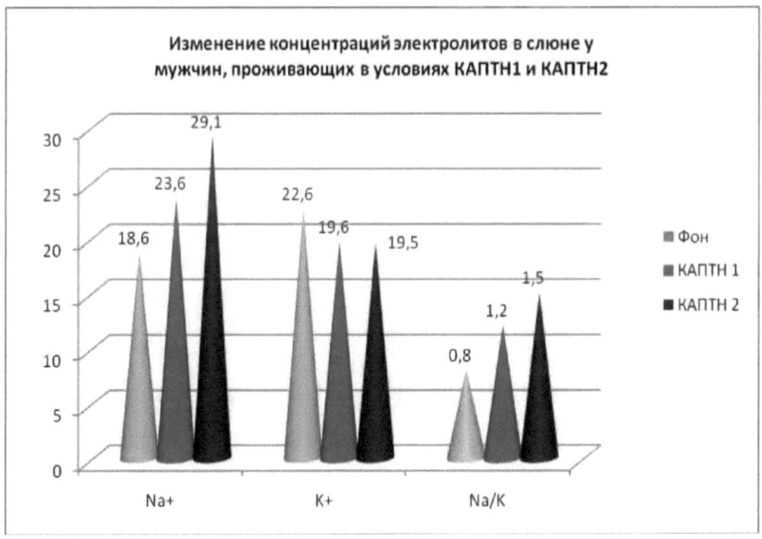

Fig. 13

The figure shows that in men living in conditions with a low rank of anthropotechnogenic load the concentration of sodium ions increases 1.3 times, and the concentration of potassium ions decreases 1.2 times. These changes are more pronounced in conditions with a high rank of anthropotechnogenic load: the concentration of sodium ions increases 1.6 times, and the concentration of potassium ions decreases 1.2 times. The ratio of sodium and potassium ions in conditions with low rank of anthropotechnogenic load in men increases respectively by 1.5 times. This indicator almost doubles in conditions with a high rank of anthropotechnogenic load.

The results of changes in sodium, potassium, Na/K ratio in saliva of women living in areas with low and high rank of anthropotechnogenic load in comparison with background indicators are reflected in Fig. 14

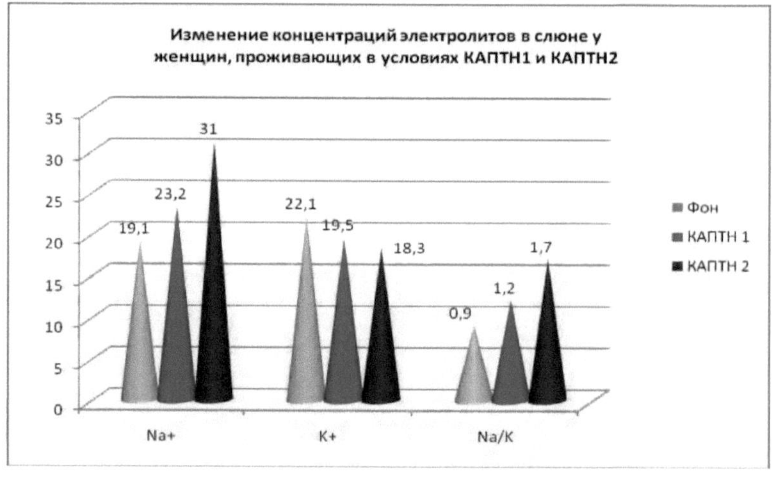

Fig. 14

The figure shows that in women living in conditions with a low rank of anthropotechnogenic load the concentration of sodium ions increases by 1.2 times, and the concentration of potassium ions decreases by 1.1 times. These changes are more pronounced in conditions with a high rank of anthropotechnogenic load: the concentration of sodium ions increases by 1.6 times, and the concentration of potassium ions decreases by 1.2 times. The ratio of sodium and potassium ions in conditions with a low

72

rank of anthropotechnogenic load in women increases respectively by 1.3 times. This indicator almost doubles in conditions with a high rank of anthropotechnogenic load.

Comparative analysis of the studied indicators in men and women shows that the concentration of sodium ions, potassium and Na/K ratio in them practically does not differ both in conditions of residence with low rank of anthropotechnogenic load and in conditions with high rank of anthropotechnogenic load. Comparison of the concentration of sodium ions, potassium ions and Na/K ratio in men living in conditions with low rank of anthropotechnogenic load with the background data shows that there is a significant increase (p<0.05) of sodium ions and Na/K ratio (1.5 times) and a decrease (p<0.05) of potassium ions. Similar changes are observed in women living in conditions with low rank of anthropotechnogenic load. These changes are more pronounced in men and women living in conditions with a high rank of anthropotechnogenic load. In men and women, sodium ion concentration increases sharply (p<0.001) from 18.6 mmol/L (men) and 19.1 mmol/L (women) to 29.1 mmol/L and 31.04 mmol/L, respectively. At the same time, potassium ion concentration decreased (p 0.05) from 22.6 mmol/L (men) and 22.1 mmol/L (women) to 19.5 and 16.3 mmol/L, respectively. Due to the above changes, there is a sharp increase in Na/K ratio. When comparing the studied indicators in men and women living in conditions with low rank of anthropotechnogenic load with those in conditions with high rank, a significant increase (p 0.001) of sodium ions is noted. The concentration of potassium ions is practically unchanged in men and insignificantly decreased in women. In this regard, Na/K ratio increases more significantly in women to 1.7 (1.4-fold) than in men to 1.5 (1.3-fold). Our analysis of changes in the concentration of electrolytes shows that there is a direct correlation between changes in the concentration of sodium, potassium and Na/K ratio in human saliva and the degree of severity of anthropotechnogenic load: the concentration of sodium ions (1.6 times), potassium (1.2 times), Na/K (1.9 times) increases in the examined persons living in the area with a high rank of anthropotechnogenic load. Na/K ratio in men and women living in areas with high anthropotechnogenic load increases (p<0.001) almost 2 times compared to background.

Thus, the analysis of the concentration of sodium, potassium ions and Na/K ratio in the saliva of a person living in the area with low and high rank of anthropotechnogenic load has revealed a number of regularities. In people living in the area with a high rank of anthropotechnogenic load sharply (p<0.01) increases the concentration of sodium ions in saliva, decreases (p<0.05) the concentration of potassium ions. At the same time in men and women living in the area with a low rank of anthropotechnogenic load, there is an increase in the concentration of sodium ions respectively 1.3 and 1.2 times, and the concentration of potassium ions decreases respectively 1.2 and 1.1 times. These changes are more pronounced in men and women living in the area with a high rank of anthropotechnogenic load: the concentration of sodium ions in men and women, increases by 1.6 times, and potassium ions decreases by 1.2 times. The change in Na/K ratio shows that in men living in areas with low and high rank of anthropotechnogenic load it increases by 1.5 and 1.9 times, respectively, and in women - by 1.3 and 1.9 times.

4.2. Changes in glucose and cortisol concentrations

The results of changes in the concentration of glucose and cortisol in saliva of men living in areas with low and high rank of

anthropotechnogenic load compared to background are reflected in Fig.
15

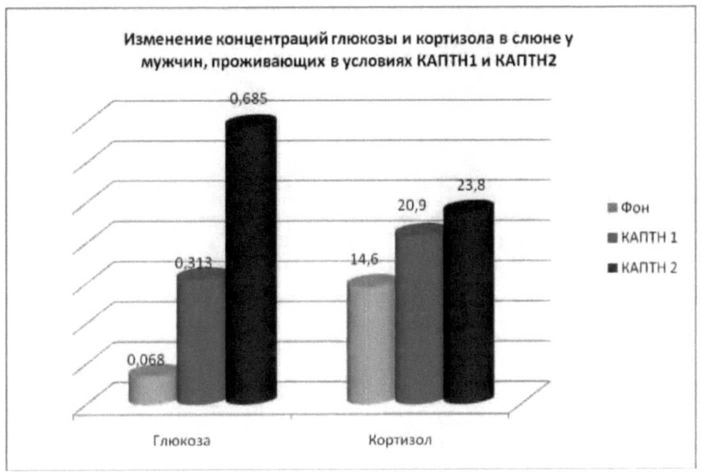

Fig. 15

The figure shows that glucose concentration increases sharply (4.6
times) in men living in conditions with a low rank of anthropotechnogenic
load. At the same time, the concentration of cortisol increases to a lesser
extent (1.4 times). These changes are more pronounced in conditions with
a high rank of anthropotechnogenic load: glucose concentration increases
10.1 times, and cortisol concentration 1.6 times.

The results of changes in the concentration of glucose and cortisol
in saliva of women living in areas with low and high rank of
anthropotechnogenic load in comparison with background are reflected in
Fig. 16

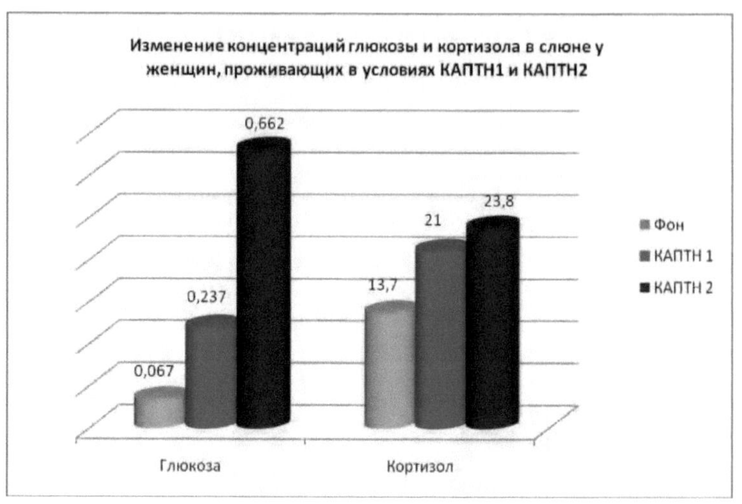

Fig. 16

The figure shows that in women living in conditions with a low rank of anthropotechnogenic load the concentration of glucose increases sharply (3.5 times). There is also a significant increase in the concentration of cortisol (1.5 times). These changes are more pronounced in conditions with a high rank of anthropotechnogenic load: glucose concentration increases by 9.9 times, and cortisol concentration - by 1.7 times. It should be noted that with increasing degree of ecopathogenic factors, the difference in the change in glucose concentration between men and women disappears. In men and women there is a sharp increase (p<0.001) in glucose concentration from 0.068 mmol/L (men) and from 0, 067 mmol/L (women) respectively to 0.685 mmol/L and 0.662 mmol/L. There is also a sharp increase in cortisol concentration (p<0.01) from 14.6 mmol/l (men) and from 13.7 mmol/l (women), respectively, to 23.8 mmol/l. When comparing the studied indicators in men and women living in conditions with low rank of anthropotechnogenic load with those in conditions with high rank, a significant increase in the concentration of glucose (p<0.001) and cortisol (p<0.05) is noted.

Thus, the analysis of glucose and cortisol concentrations in saliva of people living in the area with low and high rank of anthropotechnogenic load has revealed a number of regularities. In people living in the area with a high rank of anthropotechnogenic load sharply increases the concentration of glucose (p<0.001) and to a lesser extent increases the concentration of cortisol (p<0.01). A direct correlation between changes in the concentration of glucose and cortisol in human saliva and the severity of anthropotechnogenic load is shown: in the examined persons living in the area with a high rank of anthropotechnogenic load, the concentration of glucose (10 times) and cortisol (1.7 times) increases. In men and women living in the area with a low rank of anthropotechnogenic load, there is an increase in glucose concentration by 4.6 and 3.5 times and cortisol concentration by 1.4 and 1.5 times, respectively. These changes are more pronounced in men and women living in the area with a high rank of anthropotechnogenic load: glucose concentration in men and women increases by 10 times and cortisol concentration by 1.7 times.

Chapter 5. TYPES OF DYNAMICS OF CONCENTRATION CHANGES OF SODIUM, KALIUM, GLUCOSE, CORTIOSOL AND Na/K CONCENTRATION

Individual analysis of the concentration of sodium, potassium, glucose and cortisol ions in saliva shows their multidirectional character. In this connection, grouping people with unidirectional changes in the concentration of electrolytes, glucose and cortisol, we distinguished 4 types of their dynamics. The comparative analysis of the types of dynamics of sodium, potassium, glucose, cortisol concentration and Na/K ratio with the index of functional changes according to R.M. Baevsky allows us to correlate the revealed types of dynamics with the degree of tension of functional systems of the organism. Characterization of the obtained types of dynamics is reflected in Fig. 17

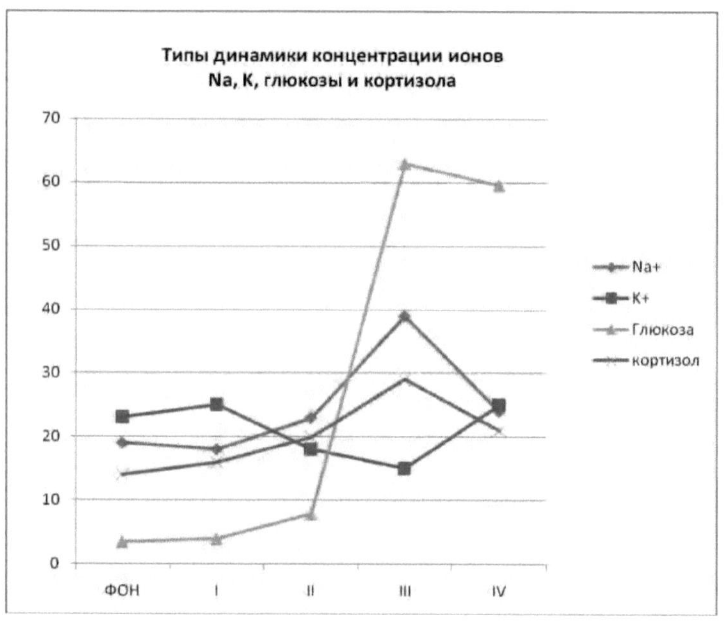

Fig. 17

These types of dynamics reflect individual features of the organism in the formation of long-term adaptation to unfavorable environmental factors. The first type of dynamics is characterized by an insignificant decrease in sodium concentration (1.1 times), increase in potassium concentration (1.1 times), decrease in Na/K ratio, insignificant increase in cortisol concentration (1.2 times) and glucose concentration (1.2 times). Persons with the first type of dynamics showed insignificant changes in the content of sodium, potassium, glucose and cortisol, which probably indicates that the revealed dynamics is within the adaptation syndrome, its initial phase, when there is a simultaneous increase in the release of adaptive hormones (adrenaline, noradrenaline, corticosteroids). This assumption is confirmed by satisfactory values of hemodynamic indices corresponding to the norm. Obviously, the experimental data indicate a high level of professional health of the examined persons belonging to this type of dynamics. This type of dynamics reflects the state of low tension of functional systems of the organism.

Biochemical indices of saliva with type II dynamics are characterized by more significant shifts in the content of the studied components. This type of dynamics is accompanied by a moderate increase in the content of sodium (1.3 times), a moderate decrease in potassium (1.3 times), an almost 2-fold increase in Na/K ratio, a significant increase in glucose concentration (2.3 times) and a slight increase in cortisol (1.4 times). This type of dynamics correspond to the state of moderate tension. Obviously, the manifestation of this type of dynamics is associated with the dissociation of hormonal release, when the production of corticosteroids is accompanied by a decrease in sympathetic-adrenal activity. The work of the cardiovascular system is characterized by insignificant changes in hemodynamic parameters. The materials of the study indicate the expenditure of adaptation reserves of the organism and the onset of the state of functional stress.

Type III of dynamics revealed during the experiment is characterized by a very wide range of changes in the content of sodium, potassium, glucose and cortisol in this type there is a significant increase in the concentration of sodium (2.1 times), a significant decrease in the concentration of potassium (1.5 times), as well as a significant increase in the concentration of cortisol (2 times) and glucose (18.5 times). This type of dynamics can be considered as an indicator of a state of high tension (sodium concentration increased, potassium concentration decreased). Changes in the quantitative composition of saliva were accompanied by a sharp deterioration of functional changes in the cardiovascular system. These phenomena can be explained by a decrease in the activity of the sympathetic-adrenal system and increased production of corticosteroids, which is characteristic of the state of dysadaptation, proceeding with the tension of regulatory mechanisms, which cannot provide the optimal mode of functioning of the organism.

In individuals belonging to the IV type of dynamics, an insignificant increase in the concentration of all studied components of saliva was noted. In this type, there is a moderate increase in the concentration of sodium (1.3 times) and a slight increase in the concentration of potassium (1.1 times) and Na/K ratio (1.3). There is a significant increase in glucose concentration (17.5-fold) and a slight increase in cortisol (1.4-fold). This type of dynamics is characterized by unidirectional changes in the concentrations of sodium and potassium and, as well as the second type, corresponds to the state of moderate tension. This type of dynamics differs from the second type by the degree of increase in glucose concentration:

in the second type glucose concentration increases 2.3 times, and in the fourth type - 17.5 times. When analyzing hemodynamic indices, no significant changes in BP and HR were found, indicating a state of satisfactory adaptation. Thus, the fourth type of dynamics was characterized by a moderate increase in sodium concentration and an insignificant increase in potassium concentration. The concentration of glucose and cortisol increased significantly. The unidirectionality of changes in sodium and potassium concentration was observed against the background of altered physiologic indices. The obtained data suggest that IV dynamics corresponds to the state of moderate tension with the corresponding character of activity. It is obvious that persons with type IV dynamics have similarity with type II in all indicators except for potassium concentration (in type II it decreases, in type IV it increases) and glucose (in type IV there is a more significant increase in glucose concentration). The manifestation of type IV dynamics, as well as the manifestation of type II, is associated with dissociation of hormonal release, when the production of corticosteroids is accompanied by a decrease in sympathetic-adrenal activity. The unidirectionality of the increase in the concentration of sodium and potassium is explained by a number of authors by the presence of probable pathologies of the gastrointestinal tract and cardiovascular system in the subjects (Kotskaya E.N., Kozlova K.T., Shkatova G.I., 1983), which is consistent with our studies.

The comparative analysis of the types of dynamics with the index of functional change shows that the I type of dynamics reflects the state of low tension of functional systems of the organism, the II type of dynamics corresponds to the state of moderate tension, the III type of dynamics can be considered as an indicator of the state of strong tension, the IV type of dynamics reflects the state of moderate tension at the corresponding character of activity.

The frequency of occurrence of the types of dynamics in men living in areas with low rank of anthropotechnogenic load is presented in Table 30.

Table 30

Types of dynamics of electrolyte composition, glucose and cortisol in saliva of men living in areas with low rank of anthropotechnogenic load

Speaker type	%%	mmol/L				
		Na^+	K^+	Na/Ka	Glucose	Cortisol
I	19.8	17.6±0.6	24.7±0.3	0.7	0.079±0.01	16.±1.2
II	64.15	23.2±0.5**	18.1±0.7**	1.3	0.156 ±0.04**	20.1±1.4***
III	9.4	39.2±1.6*	15.0±0.7*	2.6	1.26 ±0.03*	28.9±1.7*
IV	6.6	23.7±1.2**	25.0±0.1	0.9	1.19±0.02*	20.9±1.4***

* $p<0.001$; **$p<0.01$; ***$p<0.05$

Note: Significant difference of Na^+, K^+, glucose and cortisol concentrations of types II, III and IV from the first is shown

The table shows that in conditions with low rank of anthropotechnogenic load every fifth of the examined men (20%) shows the first type of dynamics of concentration of sodium ions, potassium,

Na/K ratio, glucose and cortisol. More than half of the examined men (64%) have the second type of dynamics. Only every tenth (9%) has the third type, reflecting a high degree of tension of functional systems.

The frequency of occurrence of the types of dynamics in men living in areas with high anthropotechnogenic load is presented in Table 31

Table 31

Types of dynamics of electrolyte composition, glucose and cortisol in saliva of men living in areas with high rank of anthropotechnogenic load

Speaker type	% %	mmol/L				
		Na^+	K^+	Na/K a	Glucose	Cortisol
I	9.42	18.9±0.2	23.6±0.1	0.8	0.081±0.03	16.8±1.1
II	40.6	22.9±0.3 **	19.6±0.3 **	1.2	0.131 ±0.01***	20.1±0.7 **
III	44.5	39.5±1.5 *	18.1±0.9 **	2.2	1.26 ±0.03*	29.1±1.4 *
IV	5.46	24.9±1.1 **	22.7±0.2	1.1	1.15 ±0.02*	20.3±1.2 **

* $p<0.001$; **$p<0.01$

Note: Significant difference of Na^+, K^+, glucose and cortisol concentrations of types II, III and IV from the first is shown

The table shows that the number of examined men with the first type of dynamics decreases twice (9%) and the number of examined men with the third type of dynamics increases sharply (4.7 times), amounting to about 45%.

The frequency of occurrence of the types of dynamics in women living in areas with low anthropotechnogenic load is presented in Table 32.

The table shows that in conditions with a low rank of anthropotechnogenic load every third of the examined women (29%) with the first type of dynamics, reflecting the state of low tension of functional systems of the organism. Most of the examined women (62%) with the second type of dynamics, reflecting the state of moderate tension of functional systems. Every 14th of the examined women (7%) with the third type of dynamics reflecting the state of high tension of functional systems of the organism.

Table 32

Types of dynamics of electrolyte composition, glucose and cortisol in saliva of women living in areas with low rank of anthropotechnogenic load

Speaker type	%%	mmol/L				
		Na^+	K^+	Na/ Ka	glucose	cortisol
I	29.1	16.9±0.5	25.3±0.2	0.7	0.071±0.02	17.3±0.9
II	61.8	24.1±0.2*	17.2±0.1*	1.4	0.164 ±0.02**	21.6±1.2***

| III | 7.2 | 40.7±1.2* | 14.8±0.1* | 2.8 | 1.31±0.02* | 30.7±1.1* |
| IV | 1.8 | 22.1±0.8** | 23.4±0.1** | 0.9 | 1.11±0.01* | 19.9±0.9** |

* p<0.001; **p<0.01; ***p<0.05

Note: Significant difference of Na^+, K^+, glucose and cortisol concentrations of types II, III and IV from the first is shown

The frequency of occurrence of the types of dynamics in women living in areas with high anthropotechnogenic load is presented in Table 33.

Table 33

Types of dynamics of electrolyte composition, glucose and cortisol in saliva of women living in areas with high rank of anthropotechnogenic load

Speaker type	%%	Mol/L				
		Na^+	K^+	Na/Ka	glucose	cortisol
I	8.6	16.9±0.3	26.1±0.5	0.6	0.077±0.01	17.8±1.1
II	41.3	23.2±0.1**	18.2±0.15**	1.3	0.126±0.01**	21.1±0.1**
III	44.8	41.5±1.8*	16.3±1.1*	2.6	1.22±0.02*	28.0±1.2*

| IV | 5.1 | 26.7±0.6 * | 23.8±0.1* ** | 1.1 | 1.09±0.01 * | 19.1±0.6 |

* p<0.001; **p<0.01; ***p<0.05

Note: Significant difference of Na^+, K^+, glucose and cortisol concentrations of types II, III and IV from the first is shown

The table shows that the number of examined women (9%) with the first type of dynamics sharply decreases (3.4 times) in conditions with high anthropotechnogenic load rank. At the same time, in these conditions the number of examined women with the second type of dynamics decreases (1.5 times) and the number of examined women with the third type of dynamics increases sharply (6.4 times) to 41% and 45%, respectively.

The analysis of the obtained results shows that the frequency of occurrence of electrolyte, glucose and cortisol dynamics types depends on the period of residence and the severity of ecopathogenic environmental factors. The results of the dynamics types in men with the period of residence before and after three years in areas with low and high rank of anthropotechnogenic load are presented in Fig. 18 and 19

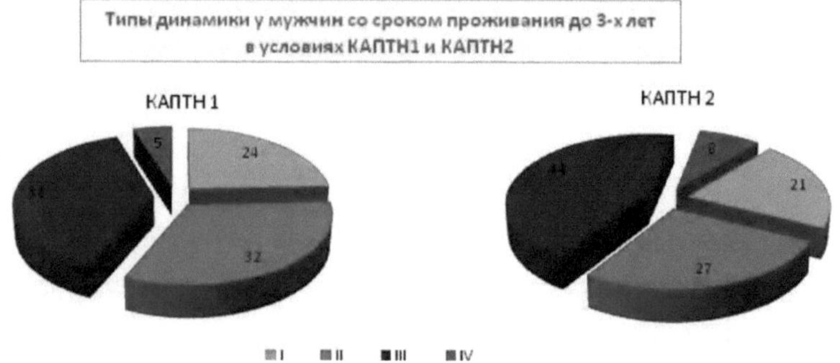

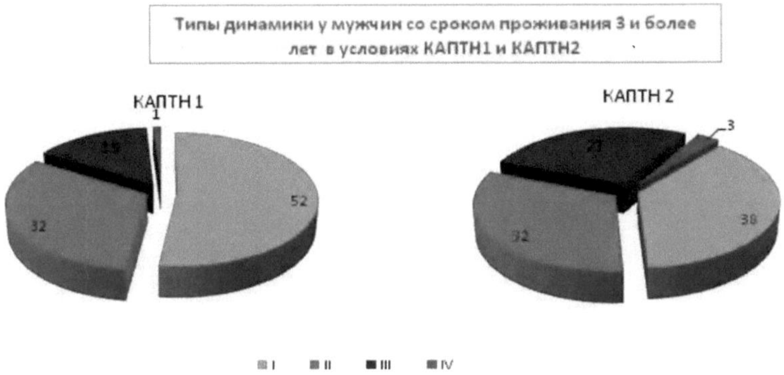

Fig. 19

The figures show that the number of persons with the first type increases significantly from 24.3% to 52.1% (2.1 times) and the number of persons with the third type decreases sharply from 37.8% to 14.5% (2.6 times), reflecting a high degree of stress of functional systems of the organism. The same regularity is observed in conditions with a high rank of anthropotechnogenic load: the number of persons with the first type increases from 20.8% to 37.5% (1.8 times) and the number of persons with the third type decreases from 43.8% to 27.5% (1.6 times). It should be noted that in men with a period of residence of more than 3 years in conditions with a high rank of anthropotechnogenic decreases the number of persons with the first type from 52.1% to 37.5% (1.4 times) and increases the number of persons with the third type from 14.5% to 27.5% (1.9 times).

The results of the types of dynamics in women with the period of residence before and after three years in areas with low and high rank of anthropotechnogenic load are presented in Figures 20 and 21

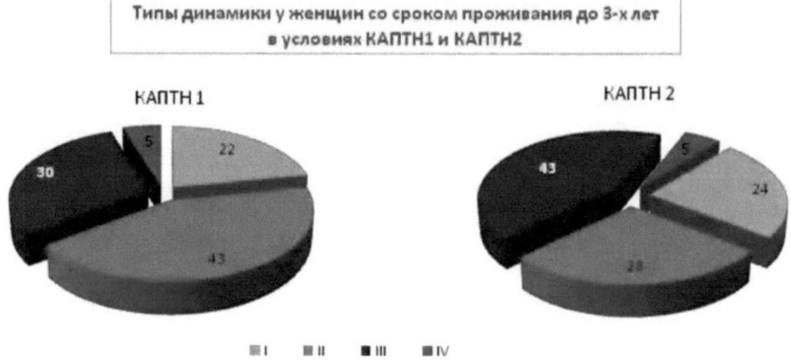

Fig. 20

Fig. 21

Our analysis shows that the number of persons with the first type significantly increases among the examined women with the period of residence of 3 and more years in conditions with low and high rank of anthropotechnogenic load: from 21.7% to 50% (2.3 times) in conditions with low rank of anthropotechnogenic load and from 23.8% to 45.9% (1.9

times) in conditions with high rank of anthropotechnogenic load. At the same time, the number of persons with the third type, reflecting a high degree of stress of functional systems of the organism, sharply decreases: from 30.43% to 12.5% (2.4 times) in conditions with a low anthropotechnogenic load rank and 42.85% to 18.9% (2.3 times) in conditions with a high anthropotechnogenic load rank.

Thus, it has been established that the frequency of occurrence of types of dynamics of electrolyte, glucose and cortisol concentrations in human saliva depends on the degree of anthropotechnogenic load and on the period of residence in the ranked territories. It follows that the types of dynamics of electrolyte, glucose and cortisol concentrations in saliva can be used as one of the objective methods for assessing human adaptation capabilities and timely prediction of prenosological and premorbid conditions arising from the inadequacy of the adaptation process.

DISCUSSION OF RESEARCH RESULTS

The study of human adaptation to changed environmental conditions remains one of the most important directions of modern ecological physiology. It is known that the objective study of individual features of human adaptation capabilities, their classification and typification are important in theoretical and applied aspects [67, 68, 35, 135, 139, 140]. To date, the criteria for assessing and predicting the effectiveness of human adaptation to changed conditions with the specification of the optimal period of living in these conditions without damage to the state of the organism in accordance with individual characteristics have not been sufficiently developed. The identification of such criteria will certainly allow for the purposeful selection of persons for various jobs in areas with high anthropotechnogenic load.

Increased rhythm of life, urbanization with its negative environmental consequences, radical socio-economic and political transformations have increased the load on life-supporting systems of the body - [5, 6].

Human professional activity is largely associated not only with the impact on the body of physical stress and nervous-emotional tension, but also with unusual environmental factors affecting its general condition, well-being and performance. Such environmental factors refer to extreme factors - to extreme and harsh environmental conditions, inadequate to the innate and acquired properties of the organism - [91]. The change of ecologically habitual habitats places increased demands on human adaptive capabilities and causes a significant restructuring of vital activity of all body systems, and under unfavorable conditions create prerequisites for the development of pathology - [3].

Extreme effects on the body affect the adaptive mechanisms, which leads to adaptation. Stress syndrome is an integral component of adaptation to all factors without exception. Its main content is excitation of higher autonomic centers and, as a consequence, activation of stress-realizing systems, the main component of which is sympathoadrenal. As a result, the effect of high concentrations of catecholamines and glucocorticoids is realized. Both of these factors have a wide range of action in the organism, the main feature of which is the mobilization of energy and structural resources of the organism - [94, 124].

When a person moves from other climatogeographic zones of habitat, in particular from the countries of the near abroad to the regions of the Russian Federation, depending on the severity of anthropotechnogenic load, contributes to a sharp change in the level of regulation of a single homeostatic mechanism and eventually failure of adaptation.

Migrant persons living in the conditions of the agro-industrial region with different ranks of anthropotechnogenic load, experience the impact of unusual environmental factors that have an unfavorable impact on his general condition, well-being and performance. Such environmental factors are referred to extreme factors, that is, extreme, harsh environmental conditions, inadequate to the innate and acquired properties of the organism - [91]. Under such conditions, the equilibration of an integral organism with the external environment is achieved only with the economical functioning of neuroendocrine regulation of the systems responsible for adaptation.

However, not always the human organism exposed to ecopathogenic factors can fully realize adaptation, which is associated with the depletion of energy and structural resources of the organism.

The totality of eco-pathogenic factors that act on a person living in a region with a high rank of anthropotechnogenic load, cause stress on the adaptation reserves of the organism, can lead to their depletion and, therefore, require careful study.

Thus, it is necessary to assess the level of health and reserve capabilities of persons living in the agro-industrial region with different ranks of anthropotechnogenic load in order to prevent the depletion of adaptive resources of the organism and the prevention of stress-related diseases. This indicates the importance of developing new, adequate methods of studying the human organism.

The earlier we can diagnose the conditions of the intermediate area between health and disease, the greater the chances of maintaining full health and active human activity. Caring for people's health and well-being requires theoretical developments and deep scientific substantiation. Health improvement of the population is closely connected with the implementation of health improvement and preventive measures, not only with the activities of medical institutions. Some aspects of these topical problems were the subject of this study.

The study of the mechanism of stress shows that stress, adaptation and health are processes dependent on each other - [125, 138]. Exposure to stress can lead to an increase in the functional reserve of the organism, which increases its health status. On the other hand, stress can lead to depletion of the body systems and the emergence of prenosological states that transition into a state of disease. The two outcomes when exposed to stress depend on the adaptive capacity of the organism, which is determined by its level of health. The task of researchers is to identify quantitative and qualitative criteria for assessing and predicting the phase of adaptation, the degree of resistance of the organism to stress with the subsequent determination of health levels.

From the many definitions of health given by Bykov A.T. et al. (2004), the following points emerge:

1. The end result of health is physical, mental and social well-being

2. Most definitions note that health is the state of being human

3. There is a direct correlation between the functional reserve of the organism, the expression of regulatory mechanisms and human health

4. health is closely related to the adaptive capabilities of the organism to changing environmental conditions

It follows from the above that the transition from health to disease occurs through a gradual decline in the human ability to adapt to changing environmental conditions with overstrain and disruption of regulatory mechanisms, which leads to changes in homeostasis and a decrease in the level of health. It should be noted that to date there is no universally accepted classification of health levels. The most all-encompassing classification is health levels by the degree of tension of regulatory mechanisms and functional reserve:

I. Individuals with satisfactory adaptation: a) optimal level of regulatory mechanisms; b) normal level of regulatory mechanisms.

II. Persons with insufficient or unsatisfactory adaptation (prenosological conditions): a) moderate tension of regulatory mechanisms; b) pronounced tension of regulatory mechanisms; c) overstrain of regulatory mechanisms.

III. Persons with disruption of adaptation, with premorbid conditions, acute and chronic diseases: a) with predominance of nonspecific changes; b) with predominance of specific changes.

The first group is characterized by the state of the organism with a sufficiently high functional reserve, in which the average fluctuation of psychophysiological, biochemical, genetic and other parameters of the organism are able to keep the living system within its morphofunctional optimum with the absence or minimally expressed tension of regulatory mechanisms. The second group is characterized by the state in which homeostasis maintenance occurs due to different degrees of expression of tension of regulatory mechanisms with increased activity of sympatho-adrenal and other systems of the organism. The third group is characterized by a decrease in the functional capabilities of the organism with the manifestation of insufficiency of protective and adaptive mechanisms and the inability of the organism to provide optimal adequate to the changed environmental conditions regulation of functional systems.

Continuous growth of scientific and socio-political information, limited time for its processing, imperfect mode of labor and rest generate disharmony in the development of personality. In the conditions of disharmony of the ratio of parameters of physiological indicators under the action of excessive stress there are tension, overstrain and failure of adaptation processes depending on the degree of such disharmony. In this regard, there is a need to develop criteria for assessing the level of stress of functional systems of the organism under stress and timely diagnosis of its inadequate impact.

It is known that stress-response is a necessary link in the formation of adaptation of the organism to environmental factors. However, in case of excessively intensive or prolonged stress-response adaptation is not formed, and stress-response leads to damage and disorders of the organism's function up to the development of a number of psychosomatic diseases. At the same time, persistent adequate adaptation to the action of any stress prevents damage and increases the organism's resistance to stress.

The action of stress can increase the functional reserve of the organism and the level of its health - in the expression of Sellier - it is eustress. In this case, the reaction of the organism proceeds without losses of the organism. On the other hand, stress can lead to depletion of the body systems, to the emergence of prenosological state, which can go into disease - this is distress. Two outcomes of stress action depend on the functional reserve of the organism, the level of health and adaptive capabilities of the organism

Currently, three degrees of functional reserve can be distinguished. Adaptation occurs due to the mobilization of functional reserves of the organism and requires a certain tension of regulatory systems. The problem of adaptation is that the "price of adaptation" did not go beyond the individual "limit", that is, did not lead to overstrain and exhaustion of regulatory mechanisms, which ultimately contributes to a decrease in the level of health. It is known that adaptation changes under the action of any stress begin with a nonspecific reaction of mobilization of functional reserves due to activation of the stress-realizing system, the main link of which is the sympathoadrenal system. The state in which the nonspecific component of the general adaptation syndrome manifests itself in the form of varying degrees of stress of regulatory systems is called prenosological - [18], in which there is a decrease in the level of health and the organism is between norm and disease. Further action of stress in this situation leads to overstrain of regulatory mechanisms, a sharp decrease in functional reserve, unsatisfactory adaptation is noted. In this state, along with nonspecific changes are more significant specific changes on the part of individual organs and systems, that is, the initial phenomena of premorbid state are noted, when changes already indicate the type of probable pathology. Thus, the manifestation of disease, which is the result of a breakdown of adaptation, is preceded by prenosological and premorbid states - [16] which are accompanied by a decrease in functional reserve and health level. At the first stages, this mechanism ensures the existence of the organism in new conditions, but it is energetically uneconomical and depends entirely on the functional reserve of the organism and its level of health. The greater the functional reserve of the organism and the higher the level of health, the greater the chances of the organism's transition to a more stable and reliable mechanism of long-term adaptation. That is, determining the adaptive capabilities of the organism, we give an assessment of health levels, which depends entirely on the functional reserve of the organism and determine its functional state.

From the above it follows that stress, adaptation and health are interdependent processes. Thus, the final result of stress and adaptive capabilities of a person is the level of his/her health.

One of the tasks of modern physiology of adaptation is the timely detection of pre- and premorbid state of the organism accompanied by a sharp decrease in functional reserve and health level. At present, there is no generally accepted methodology for diagnostics of functional reserve, health level and adaptive capabilities to stress. One of the ways to solve this problem is to assess the violation or degree of stress of regulatory systems of the integral organism. In this regard, the results of integral assessment of regulatory mechanisms of blood pressure, which characterizes the state of the cardiovascular system, can be considered reliable objective criteria. The solution of the gap in this area is possible due to the study of beta-adrenergic reactivity of erythrocyte membrane, reflecting the degree of activity of the sympathoadrenal system. An objective assessment of the state of the holistic organism can be given through the types of dynamics of the concentration of sodium, potassium, glucose and cortisol ions in human saliva.

Thus, in order to obtain comprehensive information about the state of the human body living in conditions with a high rank of anthropotechnogenic load, it is necessary to take a comprehensive approach based on modern diagnostic methods, in which a special place is given to the biochemical method of research. However, the use of biochemical methods of research in assessing the functional state of migrants living in conditions with different ranks of anthropotechnogenic load is significantly hampered by the impossibility of blood collection from a vein and finger. This necessitates the study of other human biological fluids and the development of bloodless methods that are more suitable in real-life conditions. One of the most accessible for study is saliva, and its quantitative and qualitative composition depend on the influence of various endogenous and exogenous influences on the organism - [14].

In connection with the above, it seems relevant to study the ecological and physiological peculiarities of adaptive reactions of the organism of the immigrant population of the agro-industrial region of Russia.

The aim of the present work was to study beta-adrenoreactivity of erythrocytes and the relationship between the content of cortisol, glucose, sodium and potassium ions in the saliva of the native population of Lipetsk region living in places with different anthropotechnogenic load with physiological substantiation of criteria for assessing and predicting the effectiveness of human adaptation to these conditions.

In accordance with this goal, the cardiovascular system indicators, erythrocyte membrane adrenoreactivity, as well as changes in the content of sodium, potassium, glucose and cortisol ions in saliva were studied in migrants living in conditions with different ranks of anthropotechnogenic load. The prognostic criteria for assessing the effectiveness of human adaptation in conditions with different ranks of anthropotechnogenic load for the purpose of timely prevention of depletion of adaptation resources of the organism have been developed.

The studies were conducted in the Lipetsk region in conditions with low and high rank of anthropotechnogenic load.

Among many combinations of biochemical and physiological tests, the most modern, informative and non labor-intensive ones were selected and combined into a single spectrum, and methods for their application were developed. We made a quantitative assessment of the cardiovascular system state and functional changes index, and by means of mathematical methods we analyzed the influence of the above parameters on saliva biochemistry. The complex of methods used in assessing the functional state of the contingent of subjects living in conditions with different ranks of anthropotechnogenic load allows us to identify prenosological conditions associated with the influence of eco-pathogenic factors, to predict possible health disorders.

We chose saliva as a biological fluid for the study, given that some components of its composition (namely, electrolytes sodium and potassium) are indirect indicators of the release of adaptive hormones and are most affected by stressors. In addition, the quantitative composition of other saliva components also depends on the influence of various endogenous and exogenous influences on the organism - [59]. Experiments have shown that simultaneous determination of the concentration of sodium, potassium, glucose and cortisol in saliva, as well as the study of their dynamics gives a fairly accurate and capacious representation of the functional and psychophysiological state of the subjects' organism. We chose the above biochemical components for the study based on the analysis of the significance of each of them for the human organism.

It is known that the sympatho-adrenal system is activated under any stress. One of the characteristics of the individual status of CAC is adrenoreactivity of erythrocyte membrane. In this regard, all migrants living in conditions with different ranks of anthropotechnogenic load were determined erythrocyte membrane adrenoreactivity.

Thus, the study of sensitive indicators of fundamental biological processes of the human organism at the molecular level with the help of bloodless, non-invasive methods convenient for application in the conditions of real reality was realized.

Analysis of electrolyte concentrations in saliva of men and women living in conditions with low and high rank of anthropotechnogenic load (ATN) shows that the concentration of sodium ions increases, and the concentration of potassium ions decreases. At the same time, an increase in Na/K ratio is noted. These changes are more pronounced in men and women living in conditions with a high rank of anthropotechnogenic load.

When comparing the studied indicators in men and women living in conditions with a low rank of anthropotechnogenic load with those in conditions with a high rank, a significant increase in sodium ions is noted. The concentration of potassium ions in this case in men practically does not change, and in women slightly decreases. In this regard, the Na/K ratio increases more significantly in women than in men. Our analysis of changes in the concentration of electrolytes shows that there is a direct correlation between changes in the concentration of sodium, potassium and Na/K ratio in human saliva and the degree of severity of anthropotechnogenic load.

One of the reasons for an increase in the concentration of sodium in saliva is a decrease in the total water content of the body. The main reason for the change in potassium concentration is a disturbance in the acid-base state. Potassium excretion is the result of a combination of filtration, reabsorption and secretion processes. It has been found that when the concentration of potassium in the body decreases or increases, the supply of glucose to cells is impaired.

The decrease in the activity of the subjects observed during the experiment due to weakened reflexes, hypotonia of muscles and general weakness is also a sign of potassium deficiency in the body.

Analysis of changes in glucose and cortisol concentrations in men and women living in conditions with a low rank of anthropotechnogenic load indicates their sharp increase. These changes are more pronounced in conditions with a high rank of anthropotechnogenic load. It is noteworthy that with the increase in the degree of ecopathogenic factors the difference in the change in glucose concentration between men and women disappears.

Thus, the analysis of glucose and cortisol concentration in the saliva of a person living in the area with low and high rank of anthropotechnogenic load has revealed a number of regularities. In people living in the area with a high rank of anthropotechnogenic load sharply increases the concentration of glucose and to a lesser extent increases the concentration of cortisol. A direct correlation between changes in the concentration of glucose and cortisol in human saliva and the degree of severity of anthropotechnogenic load is shown. It was noted that men and women living in the area with a low rank of anthropotechnogenic load have an increase in glucose concentration by 4.6 and 3.5 times and cortisol concentration by 1.4 and 1.5 times, respectively. These changes are more pronounced in men and women living in the area with a high rank of anthropotechnogenic load: glucose concentration in men and women increases 10 times, and cortisol concentration 1.7 times. The increase of glucose content in saliva occurs under the influence of adrenaline, which increases glucose transport from blood to saliva. In the case of rapidly increasing energy expenditure caused by heavy muscular effort, emotional excitement and factors of professional environment of damaging effect, the role of glucose in the energy of the body increases, which is explained by the rapidity of its decomposition and oxidation, as well as the fact that it is quickly extracted from the depot and can be used in extreme situations for the body.

Some authors are convinced that the blood glucose content is influenced by the cerebral cortex. The influence of the hypothalamus and the cerebral cortex on the glucose content of saliva is realized mainly through the sympathetic nervous system, which causes increased adrenaline secretion by the adrenal glands. Adrenaline also acts on the liver and muscles, causing glycogen mobilization. The glycogen reserve of muscles is used as a source of energy for their work. Also, the action of adrenaline entails an increased flow of glucose from the liver into the blood, which is used by the body during extreme physical and mental stress.

The use of indicators of cortisol content in saliva, as the results of this study show, is a convenient and reliable test for determining the degree of tension of adaptation reserves of the organism.

The increase in the concentration of cortisol in saliva can be explained by the fact that the increase in the degree of ecopathogenic factors reflexively increases the secretion of adrenaline by the brain layer of the adrenal glands. Adrenaline entering the bloodstream acts on the hypothalamus, causing the formation in some of its cells of a polypeptide - corticotropic releasing factor, which promotes the formation of adreno-corticotropic hormone in the anterior lobe of the pituitary gland. This hormone is a factor that stimulates the production of glucocorticoids in the adrenal glands. Some authors (Babsky E.B., Zubkov A.A., 1972) believe that insufficient secretion of glucocorticoids, which includes cortisol, lowers the body's resistance to various harmful influences, so we assume that the increase in the concentration of cortisol in the saliva of the examined persons is an adequate reaction of their body to the impact of negative factors of the professional environment.

Individual analysis of the concentration of sodium, potassium, glucose and cortisol ions in saliva shows their multidirectional character. In this connection, grouping people with unidirectional changes in the concentration of electrolytes, glucose and cortisol, we distinguished 4 types of their dynamics. Comparative analysis of the types of dynamics of sodium, potassium concentration, Na/K ratio, glucose and cortisol with the index of functional changes (IFI) according to R.M. Baevsky allows us to correlate the identified types of dynamics with the degree of stress of functional systems of the organism.

These types of dynamics reflect individual features of the organism in the formation of long-term adaptation to unfavorable environmental factors.

The first type of dynamics is characterized by insignificant decrease in sodium concentration, increase in potassium concentration, decrease in

Na/K ratio, insignificant increase in cortisol and glucose concentration. Insignificant changes in the content of sodium, potassium, glucose and cortisol probably indicates that the revealed dynamics is within the adaptation syndrome, its initial phase, when there is a simultaneous increase in the release of adaptive hormones (adrenaline, noradrenaline, corticosteroids). This assumption is confirmed by satisfactory values of hemodynamic indices. Obviously, the experimental data indicate a high level of professional health of the examined persons belonging to this type of dynamics. Comparison of this type of dynamics with IFI indicates a state of low tension of functional systems of the organism.

Biochemical indices of saliva with type II dynamics are characterized by more significant shifts in the content of the studied components. This type of dynamics is accompanied by a moderate increase in sodium content and a decrease in potassium level, an increase in Na/K ratio, a significant increase in glucose concentration and an insignificant increase in cortisol. This type of dynamics correspond to a state of moderate tension. Obviously, the manifestation of this type of dynamics is associated with dissociation of hormonal release, when corticosteroid production is accompanied by a decrease in sympathetic-adrenal activity. The work of the cardiovascular system is characterized by insignificant changes in hemodynamic parameters. The materials of the study indicate the expenditure of adaptation reserves of the organism and the onset of the state of functional stress.

Type III of dynamics revealed during the experiment is characterized by a very wide range of changes in the content of sodium, potassium, glucose and cortisol. In this type, there is a significant increase in the concentration of sodium and a decrease in the concentration of potassium, as well as a significant increase in the concentration of cortisol and glucose. This type of dynamics can be considered as an indicator of a state of high tension (sodium concentration increased, potassium concentration decreased). Changes in the quantitative composition of saliva were accompanied by a sharp deterioration of functional changes in the cardiovascular system. These phenomena can be explained by a decrease in the activity of the sympathetic-adrenal system and increased production of corticosteroids, which is characteristic of the state of dysadaptation, proceeding with the tension of regulatory mechanisms, which cannot provide the optimal mode of functioning of the organism. The attempt of the organism to compensate the influence of harmful environmental factors in persons with type III of dynamics of biochemical indicators of saliva is manifested in a sharp increase in the content of cortisol, which indicates a very high tension of adaptation reserves of their organism, which, in turn, is confirmed by the results of physiological indicators, which showed a mismatch of vital functions of the organism.

A similar picture in the subjects with this type of dynamics was observed in relation to glucose, the concentration of which in saliva significantly increased, indicating a sharp lack of energy reserves in the organism. Obviously, it is caused either by unformed long-term adaptation to the changed environmental conditions, or by depletion of reserve capabilities of the organism of the subjects.

The mechanism of action of glucocorticosteroids, the main one being cortisol, can probably be explained by their selective chemical reactivity. In the cytoplasm of cells of different organs there are proteins - receptors capable of selectively attaching glucocorticosteroids. The hormone then enters the nucleus, interacts with chromatin and changes the rate of transcription of certain genes. Consequently, the amount of synthesis of the corresponding proteins also changes.

The sharply pronounced changes in all the studied parameters probably reflect the onset of the state of urgent adaptation [94], which cannot provide a qualitative adaptive response of the organism to the surrounding factors.

In individuals belonging to type IV of dynamics, there was an insignificant increase in the concentration of all studied components of saliva. In this type, there is a moderate increase in the concentration of sodium and a slight increase in the concentration of potassium and Na/K ratio. There is a significant increase in glucose concentration and a slight increase in cortisol. At the same time, unidirectionality in the change of sodium and potassium concentrations is noted and, as well as the second type, corresponds to the state of moderate tension. This type of dynamics differs from the second type by the degree of increase in glucose concentration: in the second type glucose concentration increases 2.3 times, and in the fourth type - 17.5 times. When analyzing hemodynamic indices, no significant changes in BP and HR were found, indicating a state of satisfactory adaptation. Thus, the fourth type of dynamics was characterized by a moderate increase in sodium concentration and an insignificant increase in potassium concentration. The concentration of glucose and cortisol increased significantly. The obtained data suggest that IV of dynamics corresponds to the state of moderate tension with the appropriate nature of activity. It is obvious that individuals with type IV dynamics have similarity with type II in all indicators except for potassium concentration (in type II it decreases, in type IV it increases) and glucose (in type IV there is a more significant increase in glucose concentration). The manifestation of type IV dynamics, as well as the manifestation of type II, is associated with dissociation of hormonal release, when the production of corticosteroids is accompanied by a decrease in sympathetic-adrenal activity.

The frequency of occurrence of types of dynamics in men living in areas with low and high rank of anthropotechnogenic load shows that in conditions with low rank of anthropotechnogenic load every fifth of the examined men has the first type of dynamics of sodium ion concentration, potassium, Na/K ratio, glucose and cortisol. More than half of the examined men have the second type of dynamics. Only every tenth man has the third type, reflecting a high degree of tension of functional systems. In conditions with a high rank of anthropotechnogenic load, the number of examined men with the first type of dynamics decreases twice and the number of examined men with the third type of dynamics increases sharply. Analysis of the frequency of occurrence of types of dynamics in women shows that in conditions with a low rank of anthropotechnogenic load every third of the examined women with the first type of dynamics, reflecting the state of low tension of functional systems of the organism. Most of the examined women with the second type of dynamics, reflecting the state of moderate tension of functional systems. Every 14th of the examined women with the third type of dynamics, reflecting the state of high tension of functional systems of the organism. In conditions with a high rank of anthropotechnogenic load, the number of examined women with the first type of dynamics sharply decreases. At the same time, in these conditions, the number of examined women with the second type of dynamics decreases and the number of examined women with the third type of dynamics sharply increases.

The results of our studies show that the frequency of occurrence of electrolyte, glucose and cortisol dynamics types depends on the period of residence and the severity of ecopathogenic environmental factors.

Analysis of the types of dynamics in men and women with the period of residence before and after three years in areas with low and high rank of anthropotechnogenic load shows that among those examined with the period of residence of 3 and more years the number of persons with the first type increases significantly and the number of persons with the third type, reflecting a high degree of stress of functional systems of the organism, decreases sharply. The same regularity is observed among the examined persons living in areas with a high rank of anthropotechnogenic load.

Our analysis shows that the number of persons with the first type of anthropotechnogenic load increases significantly among those who have lived for 3 and more years in conditions with low and high rank of anthropotechnogenic load, and the number of persons with the third type, reflecting a high degree of stress of functional systems of the organism, decreases sharply.

Thus, it has been established that the frequency of occurrence of types of dynamics of electrolyte, glucose and cortisol concentrations in human saliva depends on the degree of anthropotechnogenic load and on the period of residence in the ranked territories. It follows that the types of dynamics of electrolyte, glucose and cortisol concentrations in saliva can be used as one of the objective methods for assessing human adaptation capabilities and timely prediction of prenosological and premorbid conditions arising from the inadequacy of the adaptation process.

The results of the conducted studies can be used in solving the issues of rationing of professional load and in the process of medical expertise in order to determine the threshold of compensatory mechanisms depending on the functional state of the organism and prediction of stability, since all the studied biochemical indicators of saliva are in close relationship and participate in the maintenance of homeostasis.

Sodium is known to be the major univalent cation of the extracellular fluid; and potassium is the major intracellular cation. Located on either side of the plasma membrane, they form a potential difference. A change in the concentration of either of these electrolytes will entail a change in the permeability of the cell membrane, which will undoubtedly have a strong influence on the metabolism of the cell and, consequently, on the metabolism of the whole organism.

Sodium, while participating in maintaining the constancy of the extracellular environment, also has a number of regulatory effects. Glucose transport into the cell directly depends on the presence of sodium in the intracellular environment: an increase in the intracellular concentration of sodium enhances the entry of glucose into the cell.

Many regulatory systems influence the maintenance of sodium and potassium concentrations in the body within narrow limits: hypothalamus, pituitary gland, adrenal glands, kidneys, right atrial wall tissue. Therefore, it is obvious that a sharp change in the content of any of these electrolytes will entail a discordance of physiological and mental functions of the body. This assumption is confirmed by biochemical indices of saliva characteristic of the examined persons with type III dynamics of the studied components. This type of dynamics, as it was already mentioned above, is accompanied by a discordance of physiological functions of the organism.

Stress syndrome is an integral component of the urgent stage of adaptation to all factors, including ecopathogenic ones, without exception. Its main content is excitation of higher autonomic centers as a consequence of adrenergic and pituitary-adrenal systems. As a result, the effect of high concentrations of catecholamines and glucocorticoids is realized. Both of these factors have a wide range of action in the organism, the main feature of which is the mobilization of energy and stressor resources of the organism.

Catecholamines increase cardiac minute volume, cause mobilization of liver glycogenic reserve and hyperglycemia, lipolysis and increase fatty acid content in blood and, consequently, increase the flow of oxygen and oxidation substrates to tissues.

Glucocorticoids act at the genetic level, activating gluconeogenesis and transamination, and thereby the conversion of amino acids to glucose, the body's structural reserve for energy.

The excess oxygen, glucose, and fatty acids resulting from the body's mobilization reactions are selectively directed to systems that carry out the increased function.

With repeated exposure of the organism to strong stimuli, the stress syndrome gradually subsides as the systemic stressor trace, which forms the basis of adaptation, is formed.

At sharp increase of ecopathogenic factors there is a lack of opportunity to realize adaptation, which is clearly manifested in the examined persons with type III dynamics of biochemical indicators of saliva. This leads to the fact that homeostasis disturbances, constituting a stress stimulus, persist for a long time. Excitation of adrenergic and pituitary-adrenal systems, constituting the content of stress, turns out to be prolonged. As a result of unusually long and intensive action of high concentrations of catecholamines and glucocorticoids a wide variety of injuries can occur, which constitute the field of so-called stressor diseases, occupying one of the main places in modern medicine.

All these facts mean that under certain conditions stress syndrome from a general non-specific link of adaptation of the organism to various environmental factors turns into a general, non-specific link of pathogenesis of diseases that limit the human life span.

It is a well-known fact in psychology and psychiatry that the state of emotional stress can persist for a long time after the elimination of the factor that caused the stress - [112]. Such post-stress activation of pituitary-adrenal and adrenergic systems, determined by emotional components of stress, plays its role in the development of stressor damage.

Therefore, in order to prevent pathologies, it is necessary to reduce the intensity and duration of the action of unfavorable eco-pathogenic factors on the body; to increase the reserves of functional systems of the body, providing its adaptive capabilities and resistance.

Thus, in the course of the conducted research the physiological features of formation of adaptive reactions of the organism in conditions with low and high rank of anthropotechnogenic load, the degree of expression of which is determined by the level of health and functional reserve of the examined persons were studied.

CONCLUSIONS.

1. As a result of the complex research on the basis of the use of various physiological and biochemical indicators with the use of modern mathematical methods of analysis, the medical and biological bases for assessing the impact of ecopathogenic environmental factors on the functional state of the human organism with the prediction of various degrees of its stress and adequacy of adaptation reactions have been developed.

2. A direct correlation between changes in the concentration of sodium, potassium, Na/K ratio, glucose and cortisol in human saliva and the severity of anthropotechnogenic load is shown: in migrants living in an area with a high rank of anthropotechnogenic load the concentration of sodium ions increases (1.6 times), potassium (1.2 times), Na/K (1.9 times), glucose (10 times) and cortisol (1.7 times).

3. Four types of dynamics of sodium, potassium, Na/K ratio, glucose and cortisol concentration in human saliva have been established, the frequency of which depends on the degree of anthropotechnogenic load. The first three types of dynamics show multidirectionality, and the fourth type shows unidirectionality of changes in the studied parameters.

4. A comparative analysis of the types of dynamics of sodium, potassium, glucose, cortisol and Na/K ratio in saliva with the index of functional changes revealed that each type reflects a certain degree of tension of the body's functional systems and its adaptive capabilities. The first type of dynamics reflects the state of low tension of functional systems of the organism (prevalence in conditions with low rank of anthropotechnogenic load is 20% among men and 29% among women, and in conditions with high rank of anthropotechnogenic load decreases

to 9%). The second type of dynamics (prevalence in conditions with a low rank of anthropotechnogenic load is 64% among men and 62% among women, and in conditions with a high rank of anthropotechnogenic load decreases to 41%) corresponds to a state of moderate tension and is associated with significant changes in the studied indicators. The third type of dynamics (prevalence in conditions with a low rank of anthropotechnogenic load is 9% among men and 7% among women, and in conditions with a high rank of anthropotechnogenic load increases to 45%) is characterized by a state of high tension of the organism and pronounced dysadaptation changes. The fourth type of dynamics (the prevalence in conditions with a low rank of anthropotechnogenic load is 7% among men and 2% among women, and in conditions with a high rank of anthropotechnogenic load is 6% among men and 5% among women) corresponds to the state of moderate tension of regulatory systems of the organism.

5.   It has been established that beta-adrenergic reactivity of erythrocyte membranes (β-ARM) provides an opportunity to assess the degree of activity of the sympathoadrenal system taking into account individual characteristics of the organism. It was noted that men living in areas with a high rank of anthropotechnogenic load experience a regular increase in the activity of the sympathoadrenal system due to the constant exposure to a combination of eco-pathogenic factors, as evidenced by a significant increase in β-ARM.

6. The results of the conducted complex research were a scientific basis for the assessment and prediction of prenosological states with the development of targeted preventive measures to prevent the depletion of adaptive capabilities of the organism under the action of a set of eco-pathogenic factors and adequate adjustment of methodological approaches

to the normalization of functional reserves of the organism and full recovery of its health.

Practical recommendations

1.   The results of the conducted research can be used in the selection of migrants traveling to work in different regions of the Russian Federation.

2.   The index of beta adrenoreactivity of erythrocytes can be used to assess the level of activity of the sympathoadrenal system during the action of stress on the body.

3.   Types of dynamics of electrolyte, cortisol and glucose concentrations in saliva can be used to assess the efficiency of human adaptation to changed environmental conditions and timely diagnosis of prenosological conditions and maladaptation phenomena (Proposal Nos. 3227/R-444; 3227/R-445).

List of references used

1.	Abarova Z.U., Shukurov F.A., Nevzorova E.V., Gulin A.V. Parameters of acid-base state of blood in the assessment of high-altitude hypoxemia //Vestnik Lipetsk State Pedagogical University. MIFE series: mathematics, information technology, physics, natural science. 2013. № 1 (4). C. 58-65.

2.	Abdulloev SA, Shukurov FA, Zoidboev ZM, Tsitsikova E.Ts. Assessment and prediction of the severity of the condition and effectiveness of treatment of patients with chronic bronchitis // Emergency physician. 2009. № 5. C. 29-30.

3.	Abdulkhakov I.U. Magnesium preparations in the practice of GPs (literature review) //Biology and Integrative Medicine 2016, 6(6), 118-132.

4. Agajanyan N.A. Ecology, health, quality of life (essays of system analysis) / Agajanyan N.A., Stupakov N.A., Ushakov I.B. - M.: AGMA, 1996. - 251 c.

5.	Aghajanyan N.A. Ethnic problems of adaptation physiology RUDN, 2007.- 57 p.

6. Agajanian N.A., Baevsky R.M., Berseneva A.P. "Problems of adaptation and the doctrine of health", M.2006 - 284 C

7. Agajanian N.A., Borisova O.I., Khlyakina O.V., Gulin A.V. Features of the development of endocrine disorders in women of reproductive age depending on the level of anthropotechnogenic load of the region of residence // Bulletin of the Ural Medical Academic Science. - 2008. - № 3. (21) - C. 28-32.

8.   Azimova M.K.. Impact of atmospheric air pollution on women's reproductive health //Biology and Integrative Medicine 2016, 1(1), 64-69.

9. Anoshkina N.L., Gulin A.V. Some aspects of health and physical development of students of a large industrial center // Medico-social problems of modern Russia. Moscow, 2008, P.10-14.

10.   Arabzoda S.N., Shukurov F.A. Activity of stress-realizing system in students in the process of their training // Bulletin of the Academy of Medical Sciences of Tajikistan. 2016. № 4. C. 19-23.

11.   Arabzoda S.N., Shukurov F.A., Kurbanov F.F. Comparative characteristics of anxiety and levels of aggression in students In the collection: Ecological and physiological problems of adaptation. Materials of XVIII All-Russian symposium with international participation. Peoples' Friendship University of Russia. 2019. C. 26-28.

12.   Arabzoda S.N., Shukurov F.A., Melikova N.H. Psychovegetative status in the assessment of adaptive capacity to emotional stress // Applied Information Aspects of Medicine. 2015. T. 18. № 1. C. 32-37.

13.   Arabzoda S.N., Halimova F.T. Comparative characteristics of mental efficiency and academic performance of students / Agajanyanov Readings - materials of the II All-Russian scientific-practical conference with international participation. Peoples' Friendship University of Russia. Moscow, 2018, 28-29

14.   Arabova Z.U., Nevzorova E.V. pH of arterial blood in humans under conditions of high-altitude hypoxemia // Bulletin of Polessky State University. - 2013. - PART 1. - P. 7-9

15.   Arabova Z.U., Nevzorova EV, Shukurov FA, Gulin AV Change in electrolyte concentrations in hypoxia // Vestnik of Tambov

University. Series: Natural and Technical Sciences. 2013. T. 18. № 6-2. C. 3283-3285.

16. Arabova Z.U., Shukurov F.A. Predicting the optimal period of human habitation at high altitudes In the collection: Ecological and physiological problems of adaptation. Materials of XVIII All-Russian symposium with international participation. Peoples' Friendship University of Russia. 2019. C. 28-30.

17. Arabova Z.U., Shukurov F.A. State of the autonomous nervous system in the assessment of human adaptation to high-mountain hypoxia // Applied Information Aspects of Medicine. 2015. T. 18. № 1. C. 73-75.

18. Arabova Z.U., Shukurov F.A., Malysheva E.V. Evaluation of oxygenation parameters in high altitude conditions // J. Vestnik of Tambov University. Series: Natural and Technical Sciences. - 2012. - Vol. 17, Vyp. 4. - C. 1282-1285.

19. Arabova Z.U., Shukurov F.A., Nevzorova E.V. Parameters of acid-base state of blood in the assessment of high-altitude hypoxemia // Bulletin of Lipetsk State Pedagogical University. - 2013 - MIFE Series, Vol. 1 (4). - C. 58-66.

20. Astashchenko A.P., Dorokhov E.V., Shukurov F.A. Study of the profile of lateral organization of sensorimotor functions in humans when performing tasks requiring increased concentration of arbitrary attention in conditions of exam stress // Avicenna Herald. 2015. № 1 (62). C. 111-115.

21. Akhmedov K.Y., Shukurov F.A. Relationship of heart rate parameters with physical performance of people during adaptation to high-mountain hypoxia // Human Physiology. 1984. T. 8. № 6. C. 943.

22. Akhmedova G.I. Features of cardiovascular disease

indicators in patients with hypothyroidism //Biology and Integrative Medicine 2020, 6(46), 140-150.\

23. Badritdinova MN, Kudratova D.Sh., Ochilova D.A. Prevalence of some components of metabolic syndrome among the female population //Biology and Integrative Medicine 2016, 2(2), 53-61.

24. Badritdinova MN, Tukhtaev DA Frequency of occurrence of risk factors of carbohydrate metabolism disorders in patients with hypertension //Biology and Integrative Medicine 2021, 5(52), 58-64.

25. Baevsky R.M. "Physiologic norm and the concept of health". Russian Physiological Journal. - 2003. - T.89, №4. - C.473-489.

26. Borisova O.I., Khlyakina O.V., Gulin A.V. Features of reproductive disorders of women living in the Lipetsk region in areas with different levels of anthropotechnogenic load // Journal of theoretical and practical medicine. - 2008a. - T 6. № 1. - C.28-31.

27. Borisova, O.I.; Khlyakina, O.V.; Gulin, A.V. Comparative ecological and physiological characterization of the significance of the reproductive function of women from the level of anthropotechnogenic load index // Avicenna Vestnik. - 2008б. - № 2. (35) - C. 113-117.

28. Bykov A.T., Malyarenko Y.E. To the question of methodological problems of health // Vestnik Restorative Medicine. - 2004. - № 1. - C. 9 - 13.

29. Vereshchak E.V., Bondar T.P. State of oxidative stress as an indicator of adaptation in gas industry workers. //Physiology of adaptations. - Volgograd, 2008. - C. 312-315.

30. Grigoriev I.V., Gritz A.N. Some possibilities that saliva presents for assessing the psycho-emotional state of a person. //Cl. lab. diagn. 2001,- № 8. -. - C. 25-28.

31.   Gulzoda K., Halimova F.T., Shukurov F.A. Ethnicity and reproductive health - a cluster-population approach to assessing reproductive health of women of fertile age LAP LAMBERT, Mauritius, 2019, 305

32.   Gulin A.V., Zasyadko K.I., Iyad Hamad S.A. Expert system for predicting students' adaptation (ESPAS) / Methodical guide. - Lipetsk, 2005. - 43 c.

33.   Gulin A.V., Shukurov F.A., Halimova F.T. Reproductive health of women of different ethnic groups //Biology and Integrative Medicine 2019, 9(37), 4-67.

34.   Davlatova D.D., Shukurov F.A., Mirzoeva Z.A., Vositzoda Z.F. Basic statistical indicators of mathematical analysis of heart rhythm in healthy people, with risk factors and in patients with arterial hypertension // Scientific and Practical Journal of TIPPMC. 2011. № 3. C. 7-9

35.   Denisov A.B. Salivary glands. Saliva. M., 2000. - 219 c.

36.   Dlusskaya I.G., Zhdanko I.M., Bogdanov Yu.V. Criterial significance of adrenoreactivity in the evaluation of some professionally important qualities of human operators // Aerospace and Environmental Medicine, - 2002.- Vol. 36, № 5.- P.12-15.

37.   Dorokhov E.V., Shukurov F.A., Semiletova V.A., Yakovlev V.N., Gorbatenko N.P. Prospects for the use of active learning methods at the Department of Normal Physiology of a medical university // Avicenna Herald. 2014. № 2 (59). C. 140-144

38.   Dubova L.I. Determination of glucose content in saliva by glucose oxidase method as an indicator of psycho-emotional stress in dentistry // Laboratory business. 1990. №4. C. 70-71.

39.   Durov A.M. Experience in the application of saliva

electrolyte studies in biorhythmological assessment of the functional state of the sympathoadrenal system in people of different age groups // Methods of mass examination. Tyumen, 1984. C. 125-126.

40.   Eliseeva E.V., Isakova L.S. Socio-psychological adaptation of IGMA students in conditions of distance learning //Biology and Integrative Medicine 2021, special issue(49), 84-89.

41.   Emelianenko S.M. Influence of intensive muscle work on some indicators of saliva of athletes // Theory and Practice of Physical Culture. - 1972. - № 2. - C. 38-41.

42.   Ermakova L.G., Kudryavtseva V.I. Assessment of the state of tension of the pilot with the help of bloodless methods of research // Military Medical Journal. 1993. №2. C. 58-60.

43.   Ermenteva L.N., Aitbaeva J.B., Akpolatova G.M. Effect of fetal cell "mediator substances" on changes in the activity of serum transaminase enzymes in rats after lethal hypobaric hypoxia //Biology and Integrative Medicine 2016, 4(4), 5-14.

44.   Zharkov AN On the heterogeneity of the response of the cardiovascular system under experimental stress. / Nikolaev V.I., Sibilev O.P. Proger E.L., Zharkov A.N., Kharitonova I.V., Belogurova E.A.// Bulletin of St. Petersburg State Medical Academy named after I.I.Mechnikov - 2005a.- № 4. - C.108-112

45.   Nikolaev V.I., Gornushkina E.Yu., Zharkov A.N. Features of the development of acute emotional stress in people depending on the strength of the excitation process in the CNS. // Man and his health SPb.: SPbMHA , 2005b. C. 190-191.

46.   Iyad Hamad. Method of assessment of adrenoreactivity of the organism by the value of - adrenoreception of erythrocyte membranes (β-ARM) to determine the level of adaptation of the student to the process of

learning in higher education. - Lipetsk: LSPU, 2004. - C.1-4.

47.   Iyad Hamad. Indicators of adrenoreactivity β - ARM in students engaged and not engaged in sports // Psychological-pedagogical and medical-biological aspects of professional training of specialists at the Faculty of Pedagogy and Psychology: Collection of scientific papers on the results of scientific and methodical work of teachers for 2003/2004 academic year. - Lipetsk, 2004. Vyp.4. - P.239-240.

48.   Karpenko V.Ya. Assessment of health, adaptation and dysaptation disorders, ways of their correction in the military border service in the North: Dissertation for a thesis. scientific degree. cand. med. sciences / V. Ya. Я. Karpenko. - N. Novgorod, 2001. - 233 c.

49.   Kodirova Sh.S. Features of treatment of psychological disorders in patients with heart disease //Biology and Integrative Medicine 2022, 1(54), 118-127.

50.   Kodirova S.S., Jabbarova M.B., Rajabova G.B. Psychosocial characteristics of patients with CHD //Biology and Integrative Medicine 2021, 4(51), 64-78.

51.   Kolpakov M.G. Mechanisms of corticosteroid regulation of body functions. Novosibirsk: Nauka, Siberian Branch, 1978. - 199 c.

52.   Komilzhanova D.K. The role of antiphospholipid syndrome in the prevention of pregnancy failure //Biology and Integrative Medicine 2017, 5(11), 21-27.

53.   Kononets I.E., Adaeva A.M., Uralieva Ch.K. Features of vegetative homeostasis and physical development of adolescents living in the low mountains of Kyrgyzstan //Biology and Integrative Medicine 2021, 6(53), 155-161.

54.   Kotelnikov VP, Morozov VN Emotional stress when working in extreme conditions // Bulletin of the Russian Academy of

Medical Sciences. - 1992. - № 11. - C. 51-57.

55.   Krasichkov D.V. Use of β-adrenoreception index of cell membranes to assess the adaptation of students depending on the state of their physical fitness // Collection of scientific works of graduate students and applicants. - Lipetsk: LSPU, 2008. - Vyp.5. - P. 177-179.

56.   Krasichkov D.V. Physiological features of adaptation of students - athletes at increased physical load in the process of learning in higher education // Abstract of dissertation, Candidate of Biological Sciences, Moscow, 2009, 22 pp.

57.   Krasichkov D.V., Gulin A.V. Functional state of cardiovascular system and adaptive capabilities of modern students / Environment and health // Collection of articles of the IV All-Russian scientific-practical conf. - Penza, 2007. - C. 117-120.

58.   Krivosheeva L.N., Sadykov F.A., Kildebekova R.N. Main risk factors of cardiovascular diseases predisposing to the formation of arterial hypertension in servicemen: Medico-social problems of modern Russia. Moscow, 2008. - C.23-27.

59.   Kuvshinov D.Yu. Arterial pressure indices at rest and under psychoemotional stress in individuals with different achievement motivation. /Physiology of adaptations. - Volgograd, 2008. - C. 254-258.

60.   Kuznetsova M.N., Pinelis V.G. Content of ions K, Na, CI and ionic Ca in salivary secretion of children. M., 1995. 8 c.

61.   Larina I.M., Whitson P., Smirnova T.M., Yu-Ming Chen. Circadian rhythms of cortisol concentration in saliva // Human Physiology. 2000. №4. C. 94-100.

62.   Leontiev V.K. Biochemical methods of research in clinical and experimental stomatology. Omsk, 1978. 89 c.

63.   Leontiev V.K., Voronin V.F. Saliva: composition, properties,

functions (Analytical review) / Central Research Institute of Stomatology. M., 2000. C. 21.

64. Medvedev V.A., Markevich O.. P. Health improvement of student youth by means of physical culture // Vysheyshaya shkola. - 2003. - № 3. - C. 72-75.

65. Meerson F.Z. Adaptation, stress and prevention. Moscow: "Nauka", 1981. 277 c.

66. Mindubaeva F.A., Shukurov F.A., Salikhova E.Y. Ethnic features of adaptive reactions of students living in different climatic and geographical conditions / In the collection: Heart rhythm and type of vegetative regulation in assessing the level of public health and functional fitness of athletes. Proceedings of the VI All-Russian symposium. 2016. C. 209-213.

67. Mukhamedova S.G., Shukurov F.A., Naimova N.M. Features of the functional activity of nephrons remaining after nephrectomy kidney in the high mountains // Reports of the Academy of Sciences of the Republic of Tajikistan. 2006. T. 49. № 6. C. 580-584.

68. Nidekker I.G., Shukurov F.A. Computer-methodology of finding the amplitude-frequency characteristics of the cardiorespiratory system in the task of adaptation to high altitude // Human Physiology. 1989. T. 16. № 6. C. 154.

69. Nikolaeva V.V., Shukurov F.A. Ethnic characteristics of growth and weight of girls in the Hissar Valley of Tajikistan //Biology and Integrative Medicine 2020, 6(46), 23-30.

70. Pavlov A.S. Psychophysiological mechanisms and consequences of daily stress. // Human Physiol. - 2002. - 28, № 4 - C. 45-53.

71. Rakhimzhanova J.A., Balkhybekova A.O., Zhyengalieva A.K., Uazirkhanov M.U. Study of autonomic balance by analyzing the cardiorhythmogram //Biology and Integrative Medicine 2021, 6(53), 240-247.

72. Savitsky V.S., Khamchiev K.M. Physiological justification of the construction of the training process of athletes sprint track cycling //Biology and Integrative Medicine 2021, 6(53),314-318.

73. Salikhova E.Y., Mindubaeva F.A., Shukurov F.A. State of regulatory systems of the body of students with different levels of motor activity // Avicenna Herald. 2012. № 1 (50). C. 125-128

74. Selje G. Essays on the adaptation syndrome. M., 1990. 254 c.

75. Sellier G. Stress without distress. / Sellier G. - M.: Progress, 1982. - 125 c.

76. Struk R.I., Dlusskaya I.G. Adrenoreactivity and cardiovascular system. Moscow: Medicine, 2003.-160 p.

77. Tananakina TP, Lysenko EA, Zadorozhny SP, Parinov RA, Kutsevol OV Comparative index assessment of the physical state of the body of young men and girls students of medical universities studying in different socio-economic conditions //Biology and Integrative Medicine 2021, 6(53), 350-358.

78. Tananakina TP, Lysenko E.A., Parinov R.A. Assessment of adaptation capabilities of young men students of medical university, studying in different socio-economic conditions //Biology and Integrative Medicine 2021, 6(53), 341-349.

79. Umbetzhanova A.T. The impact of online learning on the development of emotional intelligence in undergraduate students of a medical university //Biology and Integrative Medicine 2021, 6(53), 363-367.

80.   Fomenko L. A. Evaluation of students' psychosomatic health on the basis of mathematical and statistical modeling according to monitoring data: Dissertation for the degree of Candidate of Psychological Sciences / L. A. Fomenko. A. Fomenko. - SPb., 2002. - 195 c.

81.   Furduy F.I. - Stress, human evolution, health and sanocreatology - Scientific Proceedings of the II Congress of Physiologists of the CIS "Physiology and Human Health", Moscow-Kishineu, 2008. - C.241

82.   Furduy F.I. Problems of stress and premature biological degradation of man. Sanocreatology. Their present and future // Modern problems of physiology and sanocreatology. 2005.- C.16-36

83.   Furdui F.I., Lacusta V.N., Vudu L.F. Practical bases of sanocreatic acupuncture. Chisinau, 2007. 390 c.

84.   Habibova N.N., Avezova S.M. Characteristic features of the processes of lipid peroxidation and antioxidant activity of saliva in the oral cavity in chronic recurrent aphthous stomatitis //Biology and Integrative Medicine 2019, 3 (31), 112-121.

85.   Halimova F.T. Erythrocyte adrenoreactivity in the process of adaptation of people living in areas with low and high rank of anthropotechnogenic load //Vestnik Avicenna 2009, 3(40), 128-132.

86.   Halimova F.T. Hormonal profile in women of reproductive age of different ethnic groups / Population health - the basis of prosperity of Russia, Proceedings of the X Anniversary All-Russian scientific-practical conference with international participation. Branch of RGSU in Anapa. 2016, 322-324

87.   Halimova F.T. Thyroid and adrenal hormones in predicting the risk group of violation of women's reproductive health / Proceedings

of the XXIII Congress of the I.P. Pavlov Physiological Society with international participation, M., 2017, 201-202

88. Halimova F.T. Immuno-genetic markers of hereditary predisposition to antiphospholipid reaction //Vestnik of the Academy of Medical Sciences of Tajikistan 2017, 4(24), 78-81

89. Halimova F.T. Cluster approach to the assessment of women's reproductive health //Vestnik of the Academy of Medical Sciences of Tajikistan 2017, 2(22), 72-76

90. Halimova F.T. Hereditary predisposition to antiphospholipid reaction /Ecological and physiological problems of adaptation - materials of XVIII All-Russian symposium with international participation. Peoples' Friendship University of Russia. 2019, 239-241

91. Halimova F.T. Features of gonadotropic and thyroid hormones in women living in different climatogeographical zones / Agajanianov Readings - materials of the II All-Russian scientific-practical conference with international participation. Peoples' Friendship University of Russia. Moscow, 2018, 271-272

92. Halimova F.T. Features of antiphospholipid reaction indicators in women living in different climatogeographical zones //Vestnik of the Academy of Medical Sciences of Tajikistan 2018, 8, 1(25), 98-103

93. Halimova F.T. Features of the average regional indicators of cellular immunity in women living in different climatogeographical conditions // Vestnik of Tambov University. Series: Natural and Technical Sciences 2017, 22, 1, 217-220

94. Halimova F.T. Evaluation of thyroid system in women of different ethnic groups taking into account climatogeographical

conditions of residence //Health, Demography, Ecology of Finno-Ugric Peoples 2015, 4, 88-91

95.   Halimova F.T. Indicators of immunogenetic profile in the assessment of reproductive health of women living in different climatic and geographical zones // Bulletin of the Academy of Medical Sciences of Tajikistan 2016, 3, 114-119

96.   Halimova F.T. Population features in women of fertile age /Ecological and physiological problems of adaptation - materials of the XVII All-Russian symposium with international participation. Peoples' Friendship University of Russia. 2017, 274-275

97.   Halimova F.T. Epigenetic factors in the diagnosis of reproductive disorders //Vestnik of the Academy of Medical Sciences of Tajikistan 2017, 3(23), 91-97

98.   Khalimova F.T., Abdusattorova M.A. State of reproductive health on the indicators of cellular autoimmunity /Agadzhanyanov Readings - materials of the II All-Russian scientific-practical conference with international participation. Peoples' Friendship University of Russia. Moscow, 2018, 273-274

99.   Halimova F.T., Ganizoda M.H., Abdusattorova M.A. Immunophysiological features of reproductive health development of antiphospholipid syndrome /Ecological and physiological problems of adaptation - materials of the XVIII All-Russian symposium with international participation. Peoples' Friendship University of Russia. 2019, 241-243

100. Halimova FT, Gulin AV, Malysheva EV, Nazirova AA Clinical and laboratory characteristics of antiphospholipid syndrome in women with an obstetric history // Vestnik of Tambov University. Series: Natural and Technical Sciences 2012, 17, 4, 1285-1288

101. Halimova F.T., Gulin A.V., Malysheva E.V., Nazirova A.A. Characterization of blood coagulation parameters in antiphospholipid syndrome // Vestnik of Tambov University. Series: Natural and Technical Sciences 2102, 17, 5, 1449-1451

102. Halimova F.T., Gulin A.V., Nevzorova E.V., Nazirova A.A., Shukurov F.A. Determination of the criterion values of reproductive hormones in the formation of the risk group of reproductive disorders // Vestnik of Tambov University. Series: Natural and Technical Sciences. 2015. T. 20. № 6. C. 1640-1643.

103. Halimova F.T., Gulin A.V., Nevzorova E.V., Nazirova A.A., Shukurov F.A. Evaluation of reproductive hormonal profile in women of different ethnic groups, taking into account climatic and geographical conditions of residence // Vestnik of Tambov University. Series: Natural and Technical Sciences. 2015. T. 20. № 6. C. 1644-1648.

104. Halimova FT, Gulin AV, Nevzorova EV, Shukurov FA Ethnic peculiarities of the immunogenetic profile of women living in different climatogeographic zones // In Proceedings: Health of the population - the basis of prosperity of Russia. Materials of X Jubilee All-Russian scientific-practical conference with international participation. Branch of RGSU in Anapa. 2016. C. 325-328.

105. Halimova F.T., Gulin A.V., Shukurov F.A. Changes in the biochemical composition of saliva in people living in areas with low and high rank anthropotechnogenic load // Proceedings of the Academy of Sciences of the Republic of Tajikistan. Department of Biological and Medical Sciences. 2009. № 2. C. 59-63.

106. Halimova F.T., Gulin A.V., Shukurov F.A. Features of the average regional indicators of hormonal profile in women living in different climatogeographical conditions // Vestnik of Tambov

University. Series: Natural and Technical Sciences. 2016. T. 21. № 6. C. 2289-2294.

107. Halimova F.T., Gulin A.V., Shukurov F.A. Characterization of humoral autoimmunity in women of different ethnic groups // Health, Demography, Ecology of Finno-Ugric Peoples 2015, 4, 91-93

108. Halimova F.T., Zuhurova P.M. Genetic predisposition of students to obesity / Agajanianov Readings - materials of the II All-Russian scientific-practical conference with international participation. Peoples' Friendship University of Russia. Moscow, 2018, 274-275

109. Halimova FT, Nevzorova EV, Gulin AV, Nazirova AA Immunoreactivity of the body of women of reproductive age living in the Lipetsk region // In the World of Scientific Discoveries. 2014. № 2 (50). C. 353-359

110. Halimova F.T., Nevzorova E.V., Gulin A.V., Nazirova A.A. Determination of the regional norm of immunological parameters in women of fertile age living in the Lipetsk region // Vestnik of Tambov University. Series: Natural and Technical Sciences 2013, 18, 6-2, 3286-3288

111. Halimova F.T., Nevzorova E.V., Gulin A.V., Nazirova A.A., Shutova S.V. Characteristics of the immune status of women living in the Republic of Tajikistan / Actual problems of natural sciences - materials of the International extramural scientific-practical conference. otv. 2014, 118-123

112. Halimova FT, Nevzorova EV, Gulin AV, Shukurov FA Comparative characteristics of the immunogenetic profile of women in Tajikistan and the Central Black Earth region of Russia // Vestnik of Tambov University. Series: Natural and Technical Sciences. 2016. T. 21. № 1. C. 231-235.

113. Halimova F.T., Nevzorova E.V., Gulin A.V., Shutova S.V. Determination of lupus-type anticoagulants in the evaluation of antiphospholipid syndrome /Actual Problems of Natural Sciences 2013, 19-24

114. Halimova FT, Nevzorova EV, Shukurov FA, Gulin AV Determination of the predictive value of IGG to prothrombin in relation to the evaluation of antiphospholipid syndrome // In Proceedings: Health for All. Collection of articles of the V International Scientific and Practical Conference. Editorial Board: K.K. Shebeko [et al]. 2013. C. 267-268

115. Halimova FT, Nevzorova EV, Shukurov FA, Gulin AV Role of proteins - cofactors in the development of antiphospholipid syndrome // Vestnik of Lipetsk State Pedagogical University. Series MIFE: Mathematics, Information Technologies, Physics, Natural Science 2013, 1(4), 113-115

116. Halimova FT, Nevzorova EV, Shukurov FA, Gulin AV Comparative characterization of reproductive immunophenotype and serum immunoglobulin levels in women of different ethnic groups // Vestnik of Lipetsk State Pedagogical University. Series MIFE: Mathematics, Information Technologies, Physics, Natural Science 2015, 1(16), 115-119

117. Halimova F.T., Shukurov F.A. Hormonal status in the assessment of reproductive health disorders //Biology and Integrative Medicine 2019, 10(38), 4-12.

118. Halimova F.T., Shukurov F.A., Arabzoda S.N. Comparative characterization of different forms of aggression with anxiety, correlation rhythmograms and functional state of the body // Bulletin of the Academy of Medical Sciences of Tajikistan 2020, 10, 2(34), 196-201

119.   Halimova F.T., Shukurov F.A., Arabzoda S.N. Forms, levels and profile of aggression in students in comparison with their academic performance // Bulletin of the Academy of Medical Sciences of Tajikistan 2020, 10, 2(34), 182-187

120.   Khalimova F.T., Shukurov F.A., Gulin A.V. Immuno-endocrine aspects of reproductive health of women of different ethnic groups (literature review) // In the book: HUMAN SCIENCE - FROM AVICENNA TO MODERNITY.   Aslonova I.J., Aslonova Sh.J., Baimuradov R.R., Vorobeychik Y.N., Gulin A.V., Karomatov I.D., Mavlonov A.A., Orziev Z.M., Orzieva Sh.Z., Ochilova D.A., Porsoev J.A., Ruziev O.A., Saidov S.A., Khaidarov N.K., Khaidarova D.K., Halimova F.T., Hodjaeva D.T., Sharipova D.S., Shukurov F.A. Bukhara, 2018. C. 4-69.

121.   Halimova F.T., Shukurov F.A., Nurmatov A.A. Assessment and prediction of reproductive health of women of fertile age // Bulletin of the Academy of Medical Sciences of Tajikistan. 2019. T. 9. № 2 (30). C. 199-208

122.   Khlyakina, O.V.; Gulin, A.V. Hygienic characterization of the action of anthropogenic environmental factors on the state of health of the population of the Lipetsk region // Medico-social problems of modern Russia. Moscow, 2007. - C.92-97.

123.   Khlyakina O.V., Karsakova Y.E., Tyatenkova N.N. Influence of technogenic factors on health indicators of the inhabitants of the industrial city. / O.V.Khlyakina, //Vestnik Pomorskogo Universitet. - 2006. - №3. - C.46-49.

124.   Tsvetaeva T.V. Dynamics of biochemical indicators of saliva under the influence of unfavorable factors of industrial environment. Medico-psychological and pedagogical problems of quality of life.

Materials of the international scientific - practical conference. / Tsvetaeva T.V. - Lipetsk, 1996. - C. 50-51.

125. Tsvetaeva T.V., Gulin A.V. Dynamics of sodium, potassium, glucose and cortisol of saliva of metallurgical workers under the influence of anthropogenic factors of the professional environment // Ecology of the Central Chernozem region of the Russian Federation: scientific and technical journal. - Lipetsk. -т. 2003. - №1. - C. 20-23.

126. Shandaulov A.H., Khamchiev K.M., Alimov A.A., Bilkenov G.B. Effect of mental-emotional load on the function of external respiration in students //Biology and Integrative Medicine 2021, 6(53), 445-452.

127. Shukurov F.A. Adaptation, stress and health Mat. 49th Scientific and Practical Conf. TSMU "Adaptation, Stress, Health", Dushanbe, 2001, pp.193-204.

128. Shukurov F.A. Interpersonal relations and vegetative status in the assessment of adaptation capabilities of students // Health, demography, ecology of Finno-Ugric peoples. 2015. № 4. C. 65-68.

129. Shukurov F.A. Organization of independent work for the formation of students' motivation for lifelong learning // In the collection: Education through life: lifelong learning for sustainable development. Proceedings of the 14th international conference. 2016. C. 262-266.

130. Shukurov F.A. Assessment and prediction of human adaptation capabilities to high altitude / In the collection: Ecological and physiological problems of adaptation. Proceedings of the XVII All-Russian symposium. 2017. C. 276-277.

131. Shukurov F.A. Assessment and prediction of individual forms of human adaptation to high mountains /Mat. of I International Conf. "Chronostructure and Chronology of Reproductive Function" and

IX International Conf. "Ecological and Physiological Mechanisms of Adaptation", Moscow, 2000, p.233-235.

132. Shukurov F.A. Assessment and prediction of the effectiveness of human adaptation to high altitude / In Proceedings: Proceedings of the XXIII Congress of the I.P. Pavlov Physiological Society with international participation. 2017. C. 1503-1504.

133. Shukurov F.A. Psychoemotional state and academic performance of students in the process of their education //In the book: Agajanian Readings. Materials of II All-Russian scientific-practical conference. Dedicated to the 90th anniversary of the birth of Academician N.A. Aghajanyan. 2018. C. 303-304.

134. Shukurov F.A. Physiological substantiation of criteria for assessment and prediction of individual human adaptation to high altitude. Author's abstract of the dissertation for a doctor of medical sciences. - Moscow, 1995. - 39 c.

135. Shukurov F.A. Formation of motivation to independent work of students //Applied information aspects of medicine. 2015. T. 18. № 1. C. 22-25.

136. Shukurov F.A. Functional reserves of the organism, level of health and adaptation capabilities of the organism to the action of stress / Scientific Proceedings of the 11th Congress of Physiologists of the CIS "Physiology and Human Health" - Moscow-Kishineu, 2008 - P 214.

137. Shukurov F.A., Arabzoda S.N. Activity of the sympathoadrenal system in the assessment of adaptive capabilities of the body // In the collection: Health of the population - the basis of prosperity of Russia. Materials of X Jubilee All-Russian scientific-practical conference with international participation. Branch of RGSU in Anapa. 2016. C. 345-348

138. Shukurov F.A., Arabzoda S.N. Characterization of forms of aggression and vegetative status in the assessment of adaptive capabilities of students //Vestnik of the Academy of Medical Sciences of Tajikistan. 2018. T. 8. № 1 (25). C. 111-117.

139. Shukurov F.A., Arabova Z.U. Vegetative status in the assessment of human adaptation to high-mountain hypoxia // Bulletin of the Academy of Medical Sciences of Tajikistan. 2018. T. 8. № 1 (25). C. 118-123.

140. Shukurov F.A., Arabova Z.U. Vegetative status in the assessment of human adaptation capabilities to high altitude // J. Bulletin of the Academy of Medical Sciences of Tajikistan. - 2018. - №1 (25). - C. 121-126.

141. Shukurov F.A., Arabova Z.U. Integral indicators of heart rate variability in the assessment of human adaptation to high altitude // Bulletin of the Academy of Medical Sciences of Tajikistan. 2019. T. 9. № 1 (29). C. 89-95.

142. Shukurov F.A., Arabova Z.U. Predicting the phase of stable adaptation and prenosologic state in people with different length of residence in the high mountains // Proceedings of the National Academy of Sciences of the Kyrgyz Republic. 2019. - №4. - C. 83-87.

143. Shukurov F.A., Arabova Z.U., Arabzoda S.N. Assessment and prediction of adaptation capabilities of the student to the action of stress // Health, demography, ecology of Finno-Ugric peoples. 2015. № 4. C. 68-71.

144. Shukurov F.A., Atlasova M.H. Nonspecific resistance in students in the process of learning and emotional stress In the collection: Ecological and physiological problems of adaptation. Materials of XVIII

All-Russian symposium with international participation. Peoples' Friendship University of Russia. 2019. C. 251-253.

145. Shukurov F.A., Boboev A.A. The state of the autonomous nervous system in the assessment of health levels // Applied Information Aspects of Medicine. 2015. T. 18. № 1. C. 212-220

146. Shukurov F.A., Irgasheva D.Z. Body mass index and height-weight index in assessing the state of health of students //In the book: Agajanyanov Readings. Materials of II All-Russian scientific-practical conference. Dedicated to the 90th anniversary of the birth of Academician N.A. Aghajanyan. 2018. C. 304-306

147. Shukurov F.A., Irgasheva D.Z., Zuhurova P.M. Activity of sympathoadrenal system in the assessment of adapatational capabilities and health levels of students / In the collection: Ecological and physiological problems of adaptation. Materials of XVIII All-Russian symposium with international participation. Peoples' Friendship University of Russia. 2019. C. 253-255.

148. Shukurov FA, Melikova N.H. Motivational activity of students and the level of anxiety under emotional stress // Russian Physiological Journal named after I.M. Sechenov. I.M. Sechenov. 2004. T. 90. № 8. C. 100.

149. Shukurov F.A., Melikova N.H. State of personal and reactive anxiety in the process of learning and emotional stress // Modern problems of physiology and morphology of man and animals. Materials of the republican scientific-theoretical conf. Dushanbe, 2007. - C.101-104.

150. Shukurov F.A., Melikova N.H., Abdurakhmanova A.A. Reactive and personality anxiety of students under emotional stress. // Avicenna Bulletin 2004. № 3-4.- C. 111-118.

151. Shukurov F.A., Melikova N.H., Halimova F.T. The role of anxiety, types of perception and ways of reacting in a conflict situation in the formation of relationships of students in academic groups In the collection: Ecological and physiological problems of adaptation. Materials of XVIII All-Russian symposium with international participation. Peoples' Friendship University of Russia. 2019. С. 255-256.

152. Shukurov F.A., Mirkosimova M. Characteristics of directions of professional education and types of perception of novelty by students //In the book: Agajanyanov Readings. Materials of II All-Russian scientific-practical conference. Dedicated to the 90th anniversary of the birth of Academician N.A. Aghajanyan. 2018. С. 306-307.

153. Shukurov F.A., Nidekker I.G. Dynamic structure of heart rhythm in the process of adaptation to high-altitude hypoxia //Cosmic Biology and Aerospace Medicine. 1981. № 3. С. 28

154. Shukurov FA, Nidekker IG, Brodetskaya EE Individual characteristics of the response of the cardiorespiratory system in humans during adaptation to high altitude // Human Physiology. 1991. T. 15. № 4. С. 105.

155. Shukurov F.A., Halimova F.T. Pre-nosological states of the body //Biology and Integrative Medicine 2019, 9(37), 68-80.

156. Shukurov F.A., Halimova F.T. Normal physiology Textbook for students of medical universities / Mauritius, 2020.

157. Shukurov F.A., Halimova F.T. Evaluation of the effectiveness of independent work of students in extracurricular time / In the collection: Proceedings of the XXIII Congress of the I.P. Pavlov Physiological Society with international participation. 2017. С. 1092-1093

158. Shukurov F.A., Halimova F.T. Psychoemotional signs of stress of students in the process of learning //Biology and Integrative Medicine 2021, 6(53), 460-466.

159. Shukurov F.A., Halimova F.T. Health levels in students under emotional stress //Biology and Integrative Medicine 2021, 6(53), 467-471.

160. Shukurov F.A., Halimova F.T., Abdullaeva M.A. Analysis of the results of quality assessment of the teacher of higher education //Biology and Integrative Medicine 2019, 12(40), 119.

161. Shukurov F.A., Halimova F.T., Arabzoda S.N. Comparative characterization of different forms of aggression with anxiety, correlation rhythmograms and functional state of the body // Bulletin of the Academy of Medical Sciences of Tajikistan. 2020. T. 10. № 2 (34). C. 196-201.

162. Shukurov F.A., Halimova F.T., Arabzoda S.N. Comparative characterization of indicators of mental efficiency and academic performance of students //Biology and Integrative Medicine 2020, 3(43), 188-201.

163. Shukurov F.A., Halimova F.T., Arabzoda S.N. Degree of anxiety and emotional lability in students in the process of their education //Biology and Integrative Medicine 2020, 3(43), 202.

164. Shukurov FA, Halimova F.T., Arabova Z.U. Homeostasis indicators in short-term human adaptation to high altitude conditions and re-adaptation //Biology and Integrative Medicine 2020, 6(46), 5-22.

165. Shukurov F.A., Halimova F.T., Melikova N.H., Arabzoda S.N. Anxiety level in predicting the motivational activity of students and academic groups //Biology and Integrative Medicine 2020, 4(44), 116-130.

166. Shukurov F.A., Halimova F.T., Mirkosimova M. Comparative characteristics of adequacy of self-esteem, anxiety and types of GND in students / Agajanian readings - materials of III All-Russian scientific-practical conference with international participation. Peoples' Friendship University of Russia. Moscow, 2020, 254-256

167. Shukurov F.A., Halimova F.T., Nurmatov A.A. Assessment and prediction of reproductive health of women of fertile age //Vestnik of the Academy of Medical Sciences of Tajikistan 2019, 9, 2(30), 199-208

168. Shukurov F.A., Halimova F.T., Sultonaliev A.H. Assessment and prediction of students' adaptation capabilities to emotional stress / Agajanianov Readings - materials of the III All-Russian scientific-practical conference with international participation. Peoples' Friendship University of Russia. Moscow, 2020, 256-257

169. Shukurov FA, Halimova FT, Yasoeva M. Motivation and active methods of teaching students to study Normal Physiology //Biology and Integrative Medicine 2021, special issue(49), 257-263.

170. Ermatov N.J., Abdulkhakov I.U. Socio-hygienic assessment of the level of morbidity among different segments of the population on the materials of applications and in-depth medical examinations //Biology and Integrative Medicine 2021, 6(53), 472-488.

171. Yushkova O.I. Psychological aspects of industrial stress in labor medicine. / Yushkova O.I., Matyukhin V.V., Shardakova E.F. // Med. labor and Prom. Ecology. - 2001. - № 8. - C. 1-7.

172. Agha-Hosseini F., Dizgah I.M., Amirkhani S.. The composition of unstimulated whole saliva of healthy dental students. //J. Contemp Dent. Pract. 2006, May 1, 7(2), 104-11.

147. Andonopoulos A.P. // Brit. J. Rheumatol. - 1991. - Vol. 30. - P. 34.6-348

148. Aydin S. A comparison of ghrelin, glucose, alpha-amylase and protein levels in saliva from diabetics. //J. Biochem. Mol. Biol. 2007, Jan 31, 40(1), 29-35.

149. Bigert C., Bluhm G., Theorell T. Saliva cortisol--a new approach in noise research to study stress effects. //Int. J. Hyg. Environ. Health. 2005, 208(3), 227-230.

150. Burton R.F., Hinton J.W., Neilson E., Beastall G. Concentrations of sodium, potassium and cortisol in saliva, and self-reported chronic work stressors. //Biol. Psychol. 1996, Feb 5, 42(3), 425-438.

151. Castro M., Elias P.C., Martinelli C.E.Jr., Antonini S.R., Santiago L., Moreira A.C. Salivary cortisol as a tool for physiological studies and diagnostic strategies. //Braz. J. Med. Biol. Res. 2000, Oct., 33(10), 1171-1175.

152. Cervera R., Font J., Gomez-Puerta J.A., Espinosa G. et al; Catastrophic Antiphospholipid Syndrome Registry Project Group. Validation of the preliminary criteria for the classification of catastrophic antiphospholipid syndrome. //Ann. Rheum. Dis. 2005, Vol. 64, 1205-1209.

153. Chaudieu I., Beluche I., Norton J., Boulenger J.P., Ritchie K., Ancelin M.L.. Abnormal reactions to environmental stress in elderly persons with anxiety disorders: evidence from a population study of diurnal cortisol changes. //J. Affect. Disord. 2008, Mar., 106(3), 307-313.

154. Clow A., Thorn L., Evans P., Hucklebridge F. The awakening cortisol response: methodological issues and significance. //Stress. 2004, Mar., 7(1), 29-37.

155. Crewther B.T., Lowe T., Weatherby R.P., Gill N. Prior sprint cycling did not enhance training adaptation, but resting salivary hormones

were related to workout power and strength. //Eur. J. Appl. Physiol. 2009, Apr., 105(6), 919-927.

156. Dlusskaia I.G., Zhdan'ko I.M., Bogdanov Iu.V. [Adrenoreactivity as a criterion for the evaluation of some professionally important qualities of the human operator] //Aviakosm. [Adrenoreactivity as a criterion for the evaluation of some professionally important qualities of the human operator] //Aviakosm. Ekolog. Med. 2002, 36(5), 12-18.

157. Elloumi M., Ben Ounis O., Tabka Z., Van Praagh E., Michaux O., Lac G. Psychoendocrine and physical performance responses in male Tunisian rugby players during an international competitive season. //Aggress Behav. 2008, Nov-Dec., 34(6), 623-632.

158. Essex B., Scott L.B.; Emergency Medical Services Personnel. Chronic stress and associated coping strategies among volunteer EMS personnel. //Prehosp. Emerg. Care. 2008, Jan-Mar., 12(1), 69-75.

159. Fairchild G., van Goozen S.H., Stollery S.J., Brown J., Gardiner J., Herbert J., Goodyer I.M. Cortisol diurnal rhythm and stress reactivity in male adolescents with early-onset or adolescence-onset conduct disorder. //Biol. Psychiatry. 2008, Oct 1, 64(7), 599-606.

160. Fauvel J.P. Stress mentol ot systime cardiovisculoire // Ann. Cardiol. Et angeiol. 2002, 51, 2, 76-80.

161. Geoffroy M.C., Côté S.M., Parent S., Séguin J.R.. Daycare attendance, stress, and mental health. //Can. J. Psychiatry. 2006, Aug., 51(9), 607-615.

162. Gulzoda M., Khalimova F., Shukurov F., Gulin A.. Population and cluster approach to assessment of reproductive health of women //Georgian medical news 2017, 270, 38-45

163. Hamilton L.D., Newman M.L., Delville C.L., Delville Y.

Physiological stress response of young adults exposed to bullying during adolescence. //Physiol. Behav. 2008, Dec 15, 95(5), 617-624.

164. Hanrahan K., McCarthy A.M., Kleiber C., Lutgendorf S., Tsalikian E. Strategies for salivary cortisol collection and analysis in research with children. //Appl. Nurs. Res. 2006, May, 19(2), 95-101.

165. Hansen A.M., Blangsted A.K., Hansen E.A., Søgaard K., Sjøgaard G. Physical activity, job demand-control, perceived stress-energy, and salivary cortisol in white-collar workers. //Scand. J. Clin. Lab. Invest. 2006, 68(6), 448-458.

166. Hansen A.M., Garde A.H., Persson R. Sources of biological and methodological variation in salivary cortisol and their impact on measurement among healthy adults: a review. //Scand. J. Clin. Lab. Invest. 2008, 68(6), 448-458.

167. Harinath K., Malhotra A.S., Pal K., Prasad R., Kumar R., Sawhney R.C. Autonomic nervous system and adrenal response to cold in man at Antarctica. //Wilderness Environ. Med. 2005, Summer, 16(2), 81-91.

168. Hellhammer D.H., Wüst S., Kudielka B.M. Salivary cortisol as a biomarker in stress research. //Psychoneuroendocrinology. 2009, Feb., 34(2), 163-171.

169. Hong R.H., Yang Y.J., Kim S.Y., Lee W.Y., Hong Y.P. Determination of appropriate sampling time for job stress assessment: the salivary chromogranin A and cortisol in adult females. //J. Prev. Med. Public. Health. 2009, Jul., 42(4), 231-236.

170. Izawa S., Kim K., Akimoto T., Ahn N., Lee H., Suzuki K. Effects of cold environmental exposure and cold acclimatization on exercise-induced salivary cortisol response// Wilderness Environ. Med. 2009, Fall, 20(3), 239-243.

171. Jessop D.S., Turner-Cobb J.M. Measurement and meaning of salivary cortisol: a focus on health and disease in children //Stress. 2008, 11(1), 1-14.

172. Jurysta C., Bulur N., Oguzhan B., Satman I., Yilmaz T.M., Malaisse W.J., Sener A. Salivary glucose concentration and excretion in normal and diabetic subjects // J. Biomed. Biomed. Biotechnol. 2009, 2009:430426.

173. Kalniņa I., Toma M.M. Use of the fluorescent probe DSM in studies of the structural and functional changes of the erythrocyte membrane. //J. Fluoresc. 2004, Jan., 14(1), 41-47.

174. Irgasheva Ja., Aldybiat I., Shukurov F.A., Mirshahi M. Physiological role of bone marrow adult stem cell cd133$^+$ //Avicenna Bulletin. 2017. T. 19. № 2. C. 177-182.

175. Mindubaeva F.A., Shukurov F.A., Salikhova Y.Y, Niyazova Y.I., Ramazanov Asror Kh. Jon mechanism of functional changes in the organism of teenagers at different levels of locomotor activity //Georgian Medical News. 2015. T. 2. № 239. C. 75.

176. Shukurov F.A., Dorokhov E.V., Yakovlev V.N., Bulgakova Ya.V., Karpova A.V., Semiletova V.A. Normal physiology. Short course for english-speaking students Dushanbe, 2015

177. Kudielka B.M., Hellhammer D.H., Wüst S. Why do we respond so differently? Reviewing determinants of human salivary cortisol responses to challenge. //Psychoneuroendocrinology. 2009, Jan., 34(1), 2-18.

178. Lasikiewicz N., Hendricks H., Talbot D., Dye L. Exploration of basal diurnal salivary cortisol profiles in middle-aged adults: associations with sleep quality and metabolic parameters. //Psychoneuroendocrinology. 2008, Feb., 33(2), 143-151.

179.   Levine A., Zagoory-Sharon O., Feldman R., Lewis J.G., Weller A. Measuring cortisol in human psychobiological studies. //Physiol. Behav. 2007, Jan 30, 90(1), 43-53.

180.   Minasian S.M., Gevorkian E.S., Daian A.V., Grigorian G.G., Grigorian G.S. [Influence of mental and emotional stress on the levels of electrolytes in the saliva of senior schoolchildren] //Gig. Sanit. 2004, Jul-Aug., (4), 46-48.

181.   Minetto M.A., Lanfranco F., Tibaudi A., Baldi M., Termine A., Ghigo E.. Changes in awakening cortisol response and midnight salivary cortisol are sensitive markers of strenuous training-induced fatigue. //J. Endocrinol. Invest. 2008, Jan., 31(1), 16-24.

182.   Pico-Alfonso M.A., Mastorci F., Ceresini G., Ceda G.P., Manghi M., Pino O., Troisi A., Sgoifo A.. Acute psychosocial challenge and cardiac autonomic response in women: the role of estrogens, corticosteroids, and behavioral coping styles. //Psychoneuroendocrinology. 2007, Jun., 32(5), 451-463.

183.   Sgoifo A., Braglia F., Costoli T., Musso E., Meerlo P., Ceresini G., Troisi A. Cardiac autonomic reactivity and salivary cortisol in men and women exposed to social stressors: relationship with individual ethological profile. //Neurosci. Biobehav. Rev. 2003, Jan-Mar., 27(1-2), 179-188.

184.   Stansbury K., Harris M.L.. Individual differences in stress reactions during a peer entry episode: effects of age, temperament, approach behavior, and self-perceived peer competence. //J. Exp. Child. Psychol. 2000, May, 76(1), 50-63.

185.   Sudhaus S., Fricke B., Stachon A., Schneider S., Klein H., von Düring M., Hasenbring M. Salivary cortisol and psychological mechanisms in patients with acute versus chronic low back pain.

//Psychoneuroendocrinology. 2009, May, 34(4), 513-522.

186. Sumi D., Hayashi T., Thakur N. et al. A HMG-CoA reductase inhibitor possesses a potent anti-atherosclerotic effect other than serum lipid lowering effects - the relevance of endothelial nitric oxide synthase and superoxide anion cavenging action. //Atherosclerosis, 2001, Vol. 155, 347-357.

187. Valentino R.J., Van Bockstaele E. Convergent regulation of locus coeruleus activity as an adaptive response to stress. //Eur. J. Pharmacol. 2008, Apr 7, 583(2-3), 194-203.

188. Wirtz P.H., Siegrist J., Rimmele U., Ehlert U. Higher over commitment to work is associated with lower nor epinephrine secretion before and after acute psychosocial stress in men. //Psychoneuroendocrinology. 2008, Jan., 33(1), 92-99.

189. Wood P. Salivary steroid assays - research or routine? //Ann. Clin. Biochem. 2009, May, 46(Pt 3), 183-196.

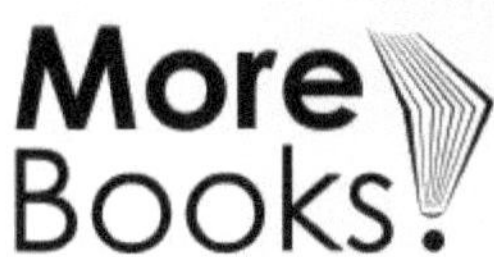

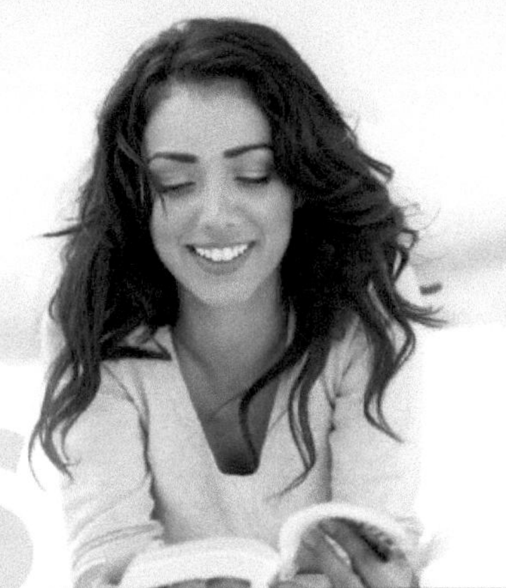

Buy your books fast and straightforward online - at one of world's fastest growing online book stores! Environmentally sound due to Print-on-Demand technologies.

Buy your books online at
www.morebooks.shop

Kaufen Sie Ihre Bücher schnell und unkompliziert online – auf einer der am schnellsten wachsenden Buchhandelsplattformen weltweit! Dank Print-On-Demand umwelt- und ressourcenschonend produzi ert.

Bücher schneller online kaufen
www.morebooks.shop

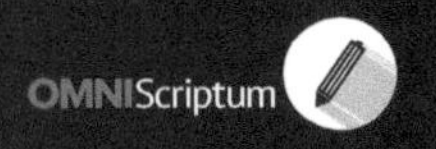

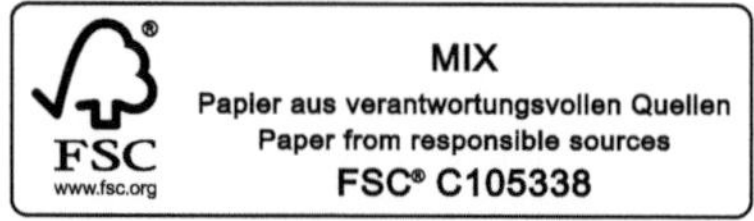

Printed by Books on Demand GmbH, Norderstedt / Germany